Bird Flu Virus: Your Personal Survival Guide

Dr Sandra Cabot

The information in this book will also be of great value to all those who suffer with
chronic infections
recurrent infections
a weakened immune system

www.whas.com.au
www.liverdoctor.com
www.weightcontroldoctor.com

Bird Flu: Your Personal Survival Guide

First Published March 2006 by WHAS Pty Ltd

WHAS Pty Ltd - Australia
P. O. Box 689, Camden NSW, 2570 Australia
Phone 02 4655 8855

SCB Inc. - United States of America
P. O. Box 5070 Glendale AZ USA 85312
Phone 623 334 3232

www.whas.com.au
www.liverdoctor.com
www.weightcontroldoctor.com

Categories - 1) Bird Flu 2) Avian Flu 3) Viral Infections 4) Fighting Infections 5) Immune System

Disclaimer - This book is NOT intended to replace or be a substitute for the care and supervision provided by your own medical doctor. At all times you should remain under the care of your doctor. The suggestions and advice in this book are to be followed only in conjunction with your regular medical care. I am not saying that I have the cure for bird flu — this book is designed to be used as a survival guide and is not a substitute for medical treatment for any flu infection.

ISBN 0975743651

Type set by Hero Productions: 0414 539 419

This book is dedicated to Nancy Beckham

Nancy Beckham died tragically in a car accident in January 2006. Nancy assisted Dr Cabot with the research of the antiviral herbs used in this book. She was a brilliant academic and research scientist. Her career as a naturopath, herbalist, homeopath, health writer and yoga teacher spanned over 25 years.

Nancy has written several books including: *Heart & Circulation, The Family Guide to Natural Therapies, The Australian Guide to Natural Therapies, Menopause - a positive approach using natural therapies, Menopause & Osteoporosis and Rejuvenation.* She also co-authored the book *Tired of not Sleeping* with Dr Sandra Cabot.

Nancy will be greatly missed by her family and myself and also by the naturopathic community and all those she has helped so much.

About The Author

Dr Sandra Cabot MBBS, DRCOG, is a medical doctor who has extensive clinical experience in holistic medicine.

Her practices are situated in Camden (phone: 02 4655 4666) and Broadway (phone: 02 9211 8624), Sydney, NSW.

Dr Sandra Cabot began studying nutritional medicine while she was a medical student and has been a pioneer in the area of holistic healing. She graduated in medicine with honours from the University of Adelaide, South Australia in 1975. During the 1980s Dr Cabot worked as a volunteer in the largest missionary Christian hospital in India, tending to the poor indigenous women.

Dr Cabot pilots herself to many cities and country towns in Australia where she is invited to speak at seminars and exhibitions.

Her free health magazines are available through health food stores and can also be read on line at www.whas.com.au and www.liverdoctor.com

Dr Cabot founded the National Health Advisory Service in 1981, as a non-government funded service. This service has provided telephone and internet advice for people of all ages who want to know all their options. Her National Health Advisory Service helps to raise money for women's refuges in Australia.

For more information phone Dr Cabot's Health Line on 02 4655 8855.

CHAPTERS . . . . Page Number

CHAPTERS . . . . Page Number

CHAPTERS . . . . Page Number

CHAPTERS . . . . Page Number

Introduction

Place: Somewhere in the Far East
Date: Sometime in the Near Future

Public health officials, heads of government and news reporters from around the world are turning their attention today to a small agricultural community on the outskirts of a prosperous Asian city, where a deadly new viral infection apparently got its start in the poultry yards that sit behind many homes and line muddy lanes.

Initial reports reveal that a severe respiratory illness first appeared here approximately four weeks ago, in people of all ages and economic status. At least 175 cases have been identified to date, with the majority of these cases showing up in the past seven days. At last count, 127 people were hospitalised, many in extremely critical condition.

Of the 31 deaths that have been reported, all are due to acute respiratory failure. The local public health agency, with the assistance of pathologists from leading research laboratories, has tested 90 percent of the infected patients and found them all to be positive for a strain of type A influenza virus never before seen in humans.

The early results from additional testing, which was still under way this morning — indicate that the majority of the viral genes originated with an avian (bird) influenza virus scientifically known as H5N1. The remainder came from a human strain of virus. This information, while widely anticipated, immediately caught the attention of health and governmental officials from all corners of the globe.

It would seem that nearly a decade after bird flu was first identified, it has finally mutated to the point that it can easily be transmitted from person to person.

As of yesterday evening, international travel into and out of this region has been banned. Quarantine measures have been put into place and all schools and public facilities, with the exception of those that are essential to daily life and maintaining health and safety, have been closed until further notice. Tens of thousands of chickens and ducks are being slaughtered.

All eyes at this point are now on neighbouring provinces and countries, in the hope that the virus has been contained locally and will not escape the immediate geographical area. Containing the bird flu is considered unlikely, though, due to the highly infectious nature of the virus, the ease with which it is now starting to spread among humans, and the fact that travel restrictions have been in place for less than 24 hours. Every high-level official contacted by this reporter is bracing for the worst-case scenario.

According to a document prepared by the World Health Organization (WHO), the virus most likely infected a significant number of visitors passing through the region prior to the quarantine and the ban on international travel. If this is indeed the case, then it won't be long until the first outbreaks are reported in other countries and on other continents. Once this occurs, there is little doubt that the crisis will rapidly intensify.

The WHO anticipates rising absenteeism in schools and businesses will quickly follow local outbreaks. Phones at health centres will be jammed with calls from concerned citizens, and the swift spread of the new virus will dominate the news and become the No. 1 topic of conversation. The public will begin clamouring for antiviral drugs and vaccinations, which will either be in very short supply or not available at all.

Soon, police and fire departments and utility companies will experience personnel shortages. Routine services will be disrupted. Hospitals and clinics will face staff shortages as doctors and nurses become ill or stay home to care for family members. All healthcare facilities will be overrun with sick and dying patients, and there will be insufficient equipment and supplies to care for anyone but the most ill.

Meanwhile, entire families will be devastated by the deaths this new strain of flu will cause. Airports will begin to close as the ranks of air traffic controllers are thinned and the majority of people become afraid to leave their homes. Trains will no longer run on schedule, or run at all. The supply chain that takes food from farms to processing plants to supermarkets and shops will begin to break down. The public will begin to hoard food and medical supplies, causing even more shortages.

Within 90 days after the first case of mutated bird flu was reported in a human, it will be confirmed: a pandemic is sweeping the world. The worst-case scenario will have arrived.

Do You Think You Will be Prepared?

Everything you just read is **hypothetical**. This **imaginary news report** is only an overview of what **might** happen if the aptly named "bird flu" virus was to mutate to the point that it could easily be transmitted between humans. And since it is truly impossible to predict the future with 100 percent accuracy, the events I have described might very well remain hypothetical for all time. Or, they could begin occurring tomorrow.

Make no mistake; bird flu is already thriving worldwide in the intestines of wild birds. And it is very contagious — and very deadly — in some domesticated birds, especially chickens and ducks. Fortunately for us, however, it hasn't developed the ability to jump from human to human. Not yet, anyway.

The question is, do you want to just wait around and see if this happens, and by doing so bet your life and the lives of your loved ones that a pandemic will never occur? Or do you want to use the practical, evidence-based knowledge found in this book to prepare yourself for a possible pandemic, and thereby significantly — ***significantly*** — improve your chances of surviving bird flu?

An influenza pandemic, which is simply a worldwide epidemic, occurs when a new flu virus to which no one has any natural immunity appears in humans, causes serious illness, and is able to spread easily from person to person and from country to country. This has happened three times in the past 100 years, and all three times the virus spread to most corners of the world within months of being detected, causing massive social and economic destruction. The most serious of these pandemics began in 1918 and is estimated to have killed as many as 50 million people worldwide before it finally ran its course.

Bird Flu: Your Personal Survival Guide was written from both a medical and naturopathic perspective to give you and your family the information you'll need to survive a global pandemic of bird flu should such an outbreak occur — and most experts agree that this is not really a matter of "if," so much as a matter of "when."

If life's daily challenges don't leave you much time for following current events, or if you are like me and occasionally discount news reports because of the tendency of some media outlets to exaggerate, then you may be wondering about now , "Is this really such a big deal? Is bird flu something I should truly be concerned about?" Unfortunately, the answer is a definite "Yes."

Viruses have always scared sensible people because of their ability to strike with no warning and kill in a matter of days, sometimes even hours. Bird flu has the potential to be one of the worst — and everyone needs to understand that there are good reasons why bird flu will kill far more people than the annual flu with which we are so familiar. When people get sick with one of the different types of flu that crop up each autumn and winter, they are partially protected by antibodies that the immune system produces from being exposed to similar flu viruses in previous years. With bird flu there will be no such immunity because our bodies have never experienced this strain of virus.

Coming down with bird flu will be like facing an enemy you think you recognise, only to discover the very moment you enter battle that this enemy is totally unknown and has tricks up its sleeve unlike any you've ever seen. Add the fact that about half of the people known to have contracted bird flu between 1997 and early 2006 didn't survive, and you have the makings of one very nasty — and extremely deadly — illness.

In **Bird Flu: Your Personal Survival Guide** I cover subjects that range from an explanation of bird flu and its origins, how bird flu spreads, the history of past pandemics, and, most importantly, how you can improve your chances of surviving an attack from bird flu by using a combination of complementary and modern-day therapies. I firmly believe that you need this "inside information" if you are going to be prepared and have a plan to survive.

It has not been an easy challenge to write this survival guide, and it has taken a lot of deep thinking on my part. I realise that it could also be controversial, as I'm dealing with an enemy that is still evolving and events that may or may not take place in the future.

There are still many bird flu questions that have no answers and a lot of problems that lack solutions.

These include:

- No natural immunity in humans to bird flu
- A shortage of antiviral drugs
- No vaccine that protects against bird flu and potential vaccine shortages
- The body's violent inflammatory response to bird flu

There are a number of books already published that discuss flu in general and bird flu in particular. My book offers a comprehensive plan for helping you to survive bird flu should the feared genetic shift take place and allow this virus to easily pass among humans. At the foundation of my survival plan, you will find good, solid research and evidence for the power of nutritional medicine.

Am I being an alarmist or premature in writing a survival plan for bird flu or a similar viral pandemic? I must answer, "NO." It is just a matter of time before we have a nasty pandemic knocking on our door.

I am not the only researcher to think this way. The British government's chief medical officer, Sir Liam Donaldson, says, "The pandemic will come. It will be real, and only if we plan can we reduce its impact."

Over the last 20 years, massive and worldwide economic, environmental and social changes have caused Mother Nature to become profoundly disturbed. We see the results in increased natural disasters, the global growth of mega-slums in big cities, and new infections and new diseases.

In many countries, particularly those that are undeveloped and poor, we have created the perfect incubator for new viruses to grow and mutate into very dangerous forms. Many millions of people in China, India, Africa and other regions of the world have deserted their farmland and crowded into cities, looking for a better life. To feed all of these people, because they can no longer raise their own food, there has been a revolution in the production of poultry and pork and other meat products. Masses of animals are crowded together in unhealthy conditions — next to masses of people living in conditions that are only marginally better. It's an ideal breeding ground for viral mutations.

We are living in a world that is growing increasingly unhealthy and where the value of local sustainable agriculture and healthy animal farming is often ignored. The bird flu virus may be another alarm clock that rudely awakens us all to the environmental dangers that many governments and industries seem to minimise.

Earlier, I asked if you'll be prepared if — when — a bird flu pandemic strikes. Don't respond to that question yet. Instead, wait and answer after you read my survival guide, when there will be no doubt about your overall knowledge of bird flu... or whether you are as prepared as you can be to survive it.

Chapter 1: Things You Need to Know and Frequently Asked Questions

If I've learned anything during my years as a doctor it is to always expect the unexpected — especially if nature is involved. As a case in point, there is Asia's disastrous tsunami of late 2004, followed just over half a year later by a chain of hurricanes that destroyed large swathes of the U.S. and Central America. Then, should nature and germs join forces, you come face to face with situations like the current emergence of avian influenza (bird flu) and its potential to become one of history's deadliest, most destructive viruses.

Tsunamis, hurricanes and similar natural disasters, while they can be predicted, cannot be controlled or prevented. Fortunately, the same is not totally true of bird flu. Though at present there is no cure for the deadly virus — either in birds or in humans — there are antiviral drugs that make the illness less severe for at least some of its human victims. My research has shown me there are also measures we can take at the personal level to either prevent this flu or lessen its seriousness. In short, sharing that information is why I wrote this book.

The media and the Internet have been filled in recent times with predictions of bird flu rapidly killing millions of people the world over, and I'd guess that many of you have given at least some thought to how you might protect your families should bird flu begin to spread rapidly in humans. I've certainly given bird flu "prevention and protection" a lot of consideration, in part because I'm a doctor and want to be in a position to help my patients. I'm also an employer of quite a few people and I want them to be protected, too. I am sure many small businesses, as well as large corporations, are making preparedness plans to keep their employees and businesses safe. Believe me; it's vitally important for everyone to do so. My home country of Australia is in close proximity to Asia — the home of bird flu — and would not be spared in a pandemic.

As I noted in the Introduction, it is possible that bird flu won't ever mutate to the point that it can easily be transmitted among humans — yet I'm someone who is not willing to bet my life or the lives of my patients on a possibility. Are you that carefree with your life? I would hope not.

In the event that avian influenza does mutate and spread, this book, **Bird Flu Virus: Your Personal Survival Guide**, provides a plan for:

- Reducing the chances of the virus infecting you
- Reducing the flu's seriousness if you do fall ill
- Knowing how to take care of yourself and keep your immune system strong so that an infection with bird flu will be more survivable

Before we get any further into "prevention and protection," however, I think it important that I answer some of the bird flu questions I've been hearing from my patients. Also, I'd like to address some of the more common misconceptions that are circulating about bird flu, and set the record straight on the disease and the most basic facts surrounding it. Since the best first step toward prevention is always knowledge — knowledge is where we'll start.

Frequently Asked Questions

I'm confused. Are bird flu and pandemic flu the same?

No. Bird flu, or avian influenza, is a group of different flu viruses that mostly infect birds, but will occasionally infect other species — most notably, humans. A flu pandemic can occur when a new subtype of flu virus emerges that has never before circulated in humans, and for which otherwise healthy people don't have any natural immunity. Avian H5N1 — the strain of bird flu virus we're always reading about — has pandemic potential since it might one day mutate to the point that it is highly contagious among humans. If this occurs, bird flu will then be considered a human flu virus, and will become a pandemic flu if it spreads around the world.

How does avian flu spread among birds?

First, it is important to understand that there are more than 100 types of bird flu, and they range from "not very contagious" to "highly contagious." Right now, the H5N1 strain is getting all of the attention for two reasons:

1. It is extremely widespread in Asia
2. A majority of the people who've had the bad luck to catch it have died

As for the larger picture, avian influenza viruses circulate among wild birds worldwide, particularly ducks and other water birds; these serve as hosts and carry the viruses in their saliva, nasal secretions and faeces. Most often the wild birds that host the viruses do not get sick, but they can and do spread the disease to susceptible birds — including domesticated birds such as chickens — through direct contact or contact with shared water or feed.

Is there anything different about the current outbreak of bird flu?

The outbreak of avian influenza we are now witnessing is the largest and the most severe on record. Never before in the history of the disease have so many countries — 18 as of this writing — been affected, with the widespread infection causing the destruction of at least 150 million mostly domesticated birds. And even with that many birds killed in order to try and halt the disease, it is thought that the earliest the flu could be under control in poultry, and this is a best-case scenario, will be sometime in 2007 or 2008. Also, there is the potential cost in human lives should this strain of bird flu evolve to the point that it can spread easily from human to human — a scary possibility at best and an extremely deadly reality at worst.

How, exactly, can or will bird flu evolve into a human flu?

According to leading experts this would most likely occur if someone already infected with a human flu virus also catches the bird flu virus at the same time. Then, the two viruses could mix their genes and form a totally new virus that has many of the same characteristics of bird flu, but with a new-found ability to spread easily among humans. This is because we won't have any built-in or natural immunity to this entirely new flu strain. The likelihood of this increases, as the avian H5N1 strain of flu spreads out of Asia and into Europe or beyond — something that unfortunately began occurring in 2005.

How are people catching bird flu now?

The H5N1 strain of bird flu, which first infected humans in Hong Kong in 1997, is caught from direct contact with infected poultry and from touching surfaces or objects that are contaminated with poultry secretions or faeces. Most cases have occurred in rural areas of Southeast Asia, where large numbers of people keep free-roaming poultry flocks that closely mingle with humans. Yet even with this constant interaction, exposure to the flu virus is most likely to occur when the infected poultry is being killed, butchered and prepared for cooking. And while there are a few cases where it's suspected that one person may have transmitted the bird flu virus to another, this can only happen at present with very close contact over a long period of time. In no case has the virus managed to spread into the community at large or even spread beyond the first generation of victims. In other words, there have been a few times when one person apparently gave bird flu to another person — but it stopped with that second person and did not spread to a third.

How many people have already caught bird flu?

As of February 2006, the World Health Organization (WHO), a United Nations agency that specialises in health, was reporting 169 laboratory-confirmed cases of H5N1 bird flu in humans since 1997, with 91 of those people dying from the disease. While this number of human cases may seem high in one sense, it is definitely low in another, as many millions of birds have been infected with the virus in some of the most heavily populated areas of the world. This just shows that, to date at least, people run a very low risk of catching the deadly virus from poultry. There are no known cases of people directly catching the H5N1 bird flu virus from wild or migratory birds.

Is it safe to travel to countries where the virus has been reported?

As of early 2006, 11 Asian nations — the Republic of Korea, Vietnam, Japan, Thailand, Cambodia, Laos, Indonesia, China, Mongolia, Taiwan and Malaysia — had reported outbreaks of bird flu in poultry, along with Russia, Kazakhstan, Turkey, Ukraine, Croatia, Romania, Iraq, Nigeria, Greece, Azerbaijan and Italy. Other countries are currently investigating outbreaks in both domestic and wild birds, so this list is likely to grow.

According to the WHO, by early 2006 human cases had been reported in seven countries: Cambodia, Indonesia, Thailand, Iraq Vietnam, China and Turkey. Most knowledgeable health authorities say — and I concur — that travel to any of these countries is safe as long as you stay away from live animal markets and poultry farms. Also, make sure you wash your hands frequently and thoroughly.

A list of bird flu affected countries can be found at
www.oie.int/downld/AVIAN%20INFLUENZA/A_AI-Asia.htm

What about eating poultry? Is that safe?

A popular misconception is that eating infected poultry, such as chicken or duck, will cause you to come down with bird flu. This is not true if the meat is fully cooked, as the virus is sensitive to heat and thorough cooking kills any and all viruses that may be present in poultry and eggs. What is true is that the bird flu virus can survive on the raw meat of infected birds, so proper hygiene such as hand washing and disinfecting all surfaces that come into contact with the raw meat is also very essential. According to information provided by the World Health Organization, there is no evidence to indicate "that any person has become infected with the H5N1 virus following the consumption of properly cooked poultry or poultry products, even in cases where the food item contained the virus prior to cooking." So, to answer the question, I'd say that it is safe to eat poultry if you handle it carefully and cook it thoroughly.

Should we expect a bird flu pandemic soon?

Honestly, nobody really knows. This is one of those questions where, as often as not, the answer depends on who you ask. In the opinion of the WHO, for instance, the risk of pandemic influenza is serious — though no timetable is mentioned. "With the H5N1 virus now firmly entrenched in large parts of Asia," says the WHO, "the risk that more human cases will occur will persist. Each additional human case gives the virus an opportunity to improve its transmissibility in humans, and thus develop into a pandemic strain. The recent spread of the virus to poultry and wild birds in new areas further broadens opportunities for human cases to occur. While neither the timing nor the severity of the next pandemic can be predicted, the probability that a pandemic will occur has increased."

Are there warning signals that will indicate a pandemic is about to start?

Without any doubt, the most important warning signal will be the appearance of bird flu in clusters of people who live in the same geographical area, and who come down with the disease in a closely related period of time. This will indicate that the virus has undergone the long-feared evolution and can be transmitted by casual human-to-human contact. Another key indicator would be a sudden outbreak of bird flu cases among healthcare workers tending to H5N1 patients. Again, this would suggest the likelihood of human-to-human transmission. In any event, I am confident that all citizens of the world with access to radio, television or the Internet would learn of a new pandemic within hours after it became official, and be in a position to very quickly take all possible precautions.

How are governments preparing for a pandemic?

This will vary greatly from country to country, of course, based on such factors as economics, vaccine-manufacturing technology and infrastructure, competency of leadership, and the amount of thought and time put into preparedness plans. Because of these limiting factors not all countries will or can be prepared. I would say that all responsible nations should at the very least be stockpiling the available antiviral medications (more about these drugs later) and considering how they will get an adequate supply of any vaccine that is ultimately produced to fight a bird flu pandemic. Because the vaccine must closely match the virus, large-scale production cannot start until the new flu has emerged and the pandemic is ongoing — and even then it could still take months to brew an effective vaccine. Governments should also be encouraging individual cities, towns and communities to plan now for how food, electricity, healthcare and other necessities will be managed during the chaos that may well accompany a pandemic.

How can I protect myself in a pandemic? What should I be doing now?

These may be the most important pandemic-related questions you can ask yourself. Because the vast majority of people will have no natural immunity (antibodies) against bird flu, the infection and illness rates will probably be extremely high. Remember, the 1918 pandemic killed as many as 50 million people worldwide. Sure, advances in medical care over the past century have given us many treatment options our ancestors didn't have. At the same time, though, transportation advances could allow the flu to spread faster and farther and circle the world in a matter of days, if not hours, instead of weeks or months. This would certainly cut down on preparation time if you weren't already prepared.

So, first and foremost, I recommend that you read and follow the comprehensive "prevention and protection" suggestions you'll find in **Bird Flu Virus: Your Personal Survival Guide**. (I did have a reason for using "survival" in the title.)

The information you'll find in my guide covers many things, and will include:

- A realistic view of bird flu and its potential to harm you and your family
- Best — and worst-case scenarios and why you need a personal survival plan
- Symptoms of bird flu and what you should do if it invades your community
- Up-to-date information on how to keep your immune system strong
- Superfoods and herbs with antiviral effects
- Minerals and vitamins that are vital for fighting the type of virus to which bird flu belongs
- Anti-flu drugs and vaccines and their pros and cons
- Proven infection control and personal protection procedures

Then, once you finish the book, share its contents with your family members and friends, but **don't lend it**—you may not have it when you really need it. Even if your national government and/or your community are not adequately prepared for a pandemic, you and the people that matter to you the most will be. This is a disease where staying informed — and being educated — may be the best defence of all and could save your life.

Chapter 2: The Flu and Past Pandemics

I had a little bird,
Its name was Enza.
I opened the window,
And in-flu-enza.

This simple rhyme, which children supposedly sang as they skipped during the flu pandemic of 1918 — is, not surprisingly, the only light-hearted comment about the flu that I can ever remember coming across. Influenza, in any of its forms, is just not a subject that people tend to make light of or joke about. And if you have ever had a bad case of the flu, I'm sure you understand why.

In my many years of practising medicine, I have seldom come across another condition or illness quite like the flu: so common, yet so misunderstood.

By definition, influenza — or "the flu"— is an "acute and highly contagious respiratory illness caused by viruses and characterised by mild to severe illness and, at times, death." There are many variations of the flu virus (see Chapter 3 for a detailed explanation), ranging from what I call the everyday or ordinary strains that each winter affect anywhere from 5 percent to 20 percent of the population, to more exotic strains such as H5N1 that are now largely confined to birds but would be deadly to people if their genetic wheels of chance ever landed on human-to-human air-borne transmission.

It's impossible to say with any accuracy when the first human (Could it have been a caveman? More than likely it was.) came down with a case of the flu. Then, as now, anyone unlucky enough to make the acquaintance of a flu virus probably suffered from a fever and headache, felt tired all of the time, and had a dry cough and a sore throat, along with a runny nose and muscle aches and pains, and maybe even an upset stomach.

The flu's very first victims likely had a rough go of it since they had not had an opportunity to acquire the natural immunity that comes with prior exposure. As generations passed, however, and as more and more people caught the flu and survived, the majority of us became at least partially immune to most of the common flu varieties. But because the H5N1 virus, the current threat, has never before crossed the species barrier from bird to human (remember: many strains of flu start in birds), almost no one on Earth has any immunity to it and all of the existing flu vaccines are practically useless against it. That's why this strain of bird flu is so lethal in humans — killing more than half of its victims to date — and that's why it's a prime pandemic concern.

Pandemics, as mentioned, are worldwide epidemics that occur when a new flu virus to which no one has any natural immunity appears in humans and spreads easily from person to person, and then spreads from country to country, until there is no place to hide and the entire human race is at risk. As best as anyone can determine, pandemics have been around for about four or five centuries now, but probably not too much longer. Why not longer? It's largely a question of transmission. It has only been in the past 500 years or so that residents of the different continents started having regular contact with one another. Prior to that, how many people travelled from Europe to Asia or from Asia to North America? Not very many…and without that person-to-person contact across vast oceans and great areas of unpopulated land, the flu simply had no way to easily spread from its region of origin.

But regardless of how far back pandemics date, it is generally the last century only that we look to for a historical perspective. I suspect that's largely because the pandemics of the past 100 years are better documented and do include the 1918 pandemic — which is considered by most experts to be the "mother of all pandemics" and the one against which modern-day pandemics will always be measured. During the 20th century, there were a total of three major flu outbreaks that are recognised as pandemics, along with several "pandemic scares." The first was the biggest: the Spanish Flu Pandemic.

1918: Spanish Flu

The 1918 pandemic, which arrived just as World War I was drawing to a close, reportedly got its name because it received more press attention in Spain than anywhere else in the world. This attention was possible because Spain was not a participant in the war and had no wartime censorship. Reputable estimates of the number of people who died worldwide from the Spanish Flu range from a low of about 20 million upward to as many as 50 million. (While there are other estimates that put the death total as high as 100 million, I do not see that a lot of credence is generally given to these.) Though the origins of Spanish Flu are not precisely known, the best guess is that it originated in China. It then spread along trade routes and shipping lanes, and was undoubtedly carried to many areas of the world by servicemen returning home from the war.

Scientists at the U.S. Centers for Disease Control and Prevention (CDC) successfully reconstructed the 1918 influenza virus, using tissue samples from infected corpses buried in cemeteries in Alaska where the ground is frozen all year round. This type of "genetic archaeology" revealed that the Spanish Flu virus was an H1N1 virus that more closely related to avian (bird) flu viruses than to influenza viruses from any other species. This indicates that a bird flu virus must have directly infected humans and adapted to them so it could spread easily between humans. Sound familiar? Ref 1, 2, 3.

To try and put the deadly nature of the 1918 pandemic in a better perspective, one writer on the subject has noted that worldwide the virus that causes AIDS killed an estimated 25 million people in its first 25 years. The Spanish Flu virus might have killed an equal number of people in only 25 weeks, beginning in September 1918. Though the statistics surrounding this pandemic do vary a bit, consider the following facts and anecdotes, which all come from reputable sources:

- The effects of the 1918 influenza pandemic were so severe that the overall death rate approached 5 percent of the world population, with an estimated 20 percent of the world population suffering from the disease.

- One story has it that four women played bridge together late into the night. By the next morning, three of them had died from influenza.
- The strain of flu was unusual in that it commonly killed many young and healthy people, as opposed to the more familiar strains of flu that generally take their victims from among the very young, the very old and the already sick.

And to give you an idea of just how far and wide the Spanish Flu virus spread, one article I read stated that the only sizeable inhabited place in the entire world with no documented outbreak of the flu in either 1918 or 1919 — when this pandemic finally died out — was the island of Marajo at the mouth of the Amazon river in Brazil.

This thoughtful take on the Spanish Flu, written toward the end of 1918, is from the *Journal of the American Medical Association:* "The 1918 has gone; a year momentous as the termination of the most cruel war in the annals of the human race; a year which marked the end at least for a time, of man's destruction of man; unfortunately a year in which developed a most fatal infectious disease causing the death of hundreds of thousands of human beings. Medical science for four-and-one-half years devoted itself to putting men on the firing line and keeping them there. Now it must turn with its whole might to combating the greatest enemy of all — infectious disease."

Unfortunately, and despite many battles won and many victories achieved, that is a war that still continues.

1957: Asian Flu

The Asian Flu was first identified in the Far East in February 1957, and was thought to have originated in northern China. Because natural immunity to this strain of flu was rare in people younger than age 65, a pandemic was predicted. Advances in technology between the pandemic of 1918 and the 1950s allowed for quick identification of the 1957 virus, and production of a vaccine was under way by May of that year.

The virus arrived in the United States by June 1957, took hold in the U.S. with a series of small outbreaks over the summer, and then began its deadly spread when school started in the autumn. This pattern was more or less repeated in many other countries as well, with school children, pregnant women, young adults and the elderly having the highest rates of infection and death. The Asian Flu pandemic ended in 1959, having killed an estimated one million to four million people worldwide.

1968: Hong Kong Flu

A few years after the Asian Flu died out, it evolved and emerged in 1968 as the Hong Kong Flu, which as the name indicates, was first detected in Hong Kong. Hong Kong Flu was milder than either of its two 20th century predecessors, with the best estimates of the worldwide death toll varying widely, ranging from a low of about 700,000 to a high of four million people.

The death toll from Hong Kong Flu was probably less than that of Asian Flu. Because it was similar to the Asian virus, many people exposed to Hong Kong Flu had previously been exposed to Asian Flu, so there was some natural immunity at work here.

1976: Swine Flu Scare

When a novel flu virus was discovered at a United States military base in 1976, it was at first labelled a "killer flu" because experts were concerned that it was related to the 1918 Spanish Flu virus and could be responsible for a similar pandemic. Further research showed that this particular virus would have been much less deadly had it ever spread — which it never did. Ultimately, the virus was named Swine Flu and was much ado about nothing, though a large-scale U.S. vaccination campaign may have contributed to the quick disappearance of this flu strain.

1977: Russian Flu Scare

In May 1977, a virus that started in northern China began to spread, causing an epidemic in children and young adults. Since this particular virus had circulated more than 20 years earlier — prior to 1957 — people born before that date were likely to have been exposed and to have developed a natural immunity against this so-called Russian Flu. By early 1978, the virus had reached most regions of the world, but because it primarily infected children, Russian Flu was not considered by experts to be a true pandemic.

2003: SARS Scare

Though similar in many ways to the flu — including its early symptoms — SARS, or Severe Acute Respiratory Syndrome, is a severe form of pneumonia that originated in southern China in 2002. It was caused by a previously unknown coronavirus, one of a group of viruses responsible for upper-respiratory illness in humans and associated with various diseases in animals.

By early 2003, SARS had spread to more than two dozen countries in North America, South America, Europe and Asia via travellers on international flights, and was recognised as a global threat. A prompt and collaborative response from international healthcare agencies was able to contain the virus, with only slightly more than 8,000 people worldwide becoming sick and just 774 SARS-related deaths.

What Next?

It should be pretty apparent by now why pandemics are such dreaded events. Once started, they can be nearly impossible to stop and it is now thought that the next full-blown pandemic could affect up to 25 percent to 35 percent of the world's population — resulting in millions of deaths, an overwhelming of health services, an interruption of many other services essential to public well being, and social and economic disruptions. A worst-case extrapolation from the toll of the 1918 Spanish Flu says a pandemic of similar seriousness could today kill up to 150 million people worldwide. That's not likely, but any way you look at it, it's not a pretty picture, either!

In one sense, if or when the next pandemic occurs, the fate of the world and the fate of your family could hang on how well governments are prepared and how well you are prepared. What our governments do or don't do is largely out of our hands, and many so-called experts might tell you that you cannot do very much at this stage to protect yourself and your family. Don't believe them. As you will read and discover in the coming pages of **Bird Flu: Your Personal Survival Guide**, there are many practical steps that can be taken now to increase your chances of survival should a bird flu pandemic occur — and I'm here to help you and tell you there is no better time to get started than the present.

Chapter 3: Understanding Bird Flu

influenza *(in floo-en za) — An acute and contagious respiratory infection that is characterised by the sudden onset of fever, chills, headache, myalgia (muscle pain) and sometimes prostration (absolute exhaustion). Cough and sore throat are common. It is usually more prevalent in the winter and the spring, and has an incubation period of one to three days. Influenza ordinarily lasts from four to seven days and may terminate by speedy lysis (you begin to feel better very quickly) or by crisis (you're in big trouble now).*

To the majority of people, it is simply "the flu." If you're a bit more formal you might instead use "influenza." As far as I'm concerned, the flu by any name is still going to be a troublesome, nasty virus that will probably be with us for as long as the sun rises in the morning and life exists on planet earth. I once read that an infectious disease specialist was asked, "If you had to rank the flu against all of the other diseases that could cause a medical apocalypse, where would it rank?"

"The flu," he replied, "would be numbers 1 through 10."

Viruses and How They Work

Viruses are very small particles—approximately one-millionth of a centimetre (2.54 cm equals 1 inch) in size — that are responsible for a wide range of illnesses, from AIDS, glandular fever, warts, cold sores and colds to hepatitis and ... you guessed it ... the flu. They also vary widely in how they look. Some viruses resemble a popcorn ball. Others may remind you of a spider or an alien spacecraft. The flu virus looks like a ball covered in spikes.

Flu viruses — and indeed, all types of viruses — are essentially parasites, in that they cannot function on their own. To live and to reproduce, a virus must find a host cell (human, animal or plant) that it can attach itself to, much like a burr sticks to your pants leg when you're out walking in the bush. Once it grabs hold, the virus will infect the host cell with its genetic material, and those genes will take over the cell and force it to make more viruses. In essence, your cell is taken hostage and turned into a virus factory.

The newly formed viruses will be released by the infected cell and drift off to infect other innocent cells. Meanwhile, the infected cells can't function properly and often die. If it happens to be your cells that are hosting the virus and your cells that are being destroyed, then you, too, might not function properly, and you, too, might die.

The actual process is much more complicated than this, of course, and involves proteins, enzymes and DNA and RNA and so forth and so on. But what's important to remember here is that a single influenza virus can produce many thousands of new flu viruses in less than a day's time, which is why people have been known to feel just fine at dinnertime, yet be dead from the flu by morning.

Influenza Type A Virus

Influenza type A viruses can infect people, birds, pigs, horses, seals, whales and other types of animals, though wild birds are the natural hosts for these viruses. Typically, wild birds do not become sick when they are infected with influenza A viruses, but domestic poultry, such as turkeys and chickens, can become very sick and die from avian influenza. But that's "typically," as some influenza A viruses do cause serious disease and death in wild birds.

Influenza type A viruses are divided into **subtypes** based on two proteins that are found on the surface of the virus.

These proteins are:

- Haemagglutinin (HA)
- Neuraminidase (NA)

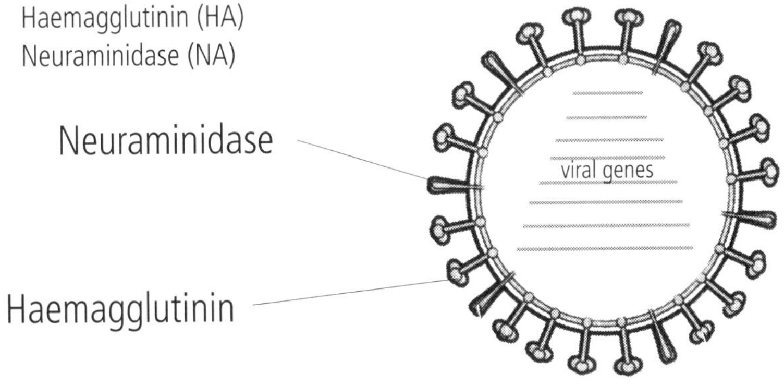

Diagram of influenza virus

According to the U.S. Centers for Disease Control and Prevention (CDC), there are 16 known HA subtypes of the influenza A virus, along with nine NA subtypes. Many different combinations of HA and NA proteins are possible. As an example, influenza A subtypes H1N1, H1N2 and H3N2 are currently in general circulation among humans. Two other subtypes, H7N7 and H3N8, cause illness in horses, with H3N8 also thought to cause illness in dogs.

Subtypes of influenza A virus are named according to their HA and NA proteins. For instance, H5N1 — which you might recognise as our newest enemy, the bird flu — is an influenza A virus with an HA 5 protein and an NA 1 protein. Got that? It's important, I think, to understand how the H5N1 bird flu virus came by its name...but I promise that from here on out, there will be no more of these complicated explanations.

Influenza Type B Virus

Influenza B viruses are usually found in humans only. Influenza type B viruses can cause illness and even death in humans, though in general they are associated with less severe epidemics than influenza A viruses and to date have not been responsible for any pandemics.

Influenza Type C Virus

Influenza type C viruses may cause mild illness in humans, but are not known to cause epidemics or pandemics.

Viral Strains

Influenza B viruses and subtypes of influenza A virus are also identified by strains, and there are many different strains of both. New strains of flu viruses appear quite often to replace older strains, through a process known as antigenic drift (more about this in a moment). When a new strain of human flu virus emerges, the antibody protection that you may have developed after being exposed to or vaccinated with an older strain might not work against the new strain. For this reason, the influenza vaccine used to fight ordinary strains of flu is updated each year to keep up with changes in flu viruses.

Drift and Shift of a Virus

Influenza viruses are continuously evolving, which means that they keep changing their genetic structure — and are great survivors for this reason. Rapidly and continually changing viruses have been described by some experts as "disguise artists" or "chameleons." No wonder our immune system has trouble recognising them and fighting them!

Viruses can change in two different ways:

- Antigenic drift
- Antigenic shift

For simplicity's sake, we'll just call them drift and shift.

- **Drift** refers to small, gradual changes that happen continually over time, to produce new virus strains that may not be recognised by antibodies to earlier flu strains. Generally, one or two of the three virus strains in the ordinary flu vaccine are updated each year to match the changes in the circulating influenza viruses.
- **Shift** is an abrupt, major change that produces a new influenza A virus not seen in humans in many years, if ever. This new virus can spread easily and cause serious disease since there is no natural immunity. Shift can occur either through direct animal-to-human transmission of a new influenza A subtype or the mixing of human and animal influenza virus genes in a human to create the new virus.

If you have followed me this far, then congratulations — you know more about the types, subtypes and strains of flu and how they drift and shift than 99.9 percent of the people in the world. Of particular concern at the present time is the H5N1 virus — the increasingly infamous bird flu.

Although avian influenza A viruses generally do not infect humans, H5N1 has shown it can do just that, primarily through direct contact with infected poultry or with contaminated surfaces such as countertops and cutting boards, but occasionally through very close contact with an infected person. Yet a lot remains, unknown about how the different subtypes and strains of avian flu virus could affect humans.

Another unknown is why the H5N1flu virus appears to thrive in the cooler months (beginning of autumn to end of winter). This just happens to match the seasonal peak for all of the common human flu viruses, and is a matter of considerable concern.

The reality that both human and avian flu viruses thrive during the same time frame is most disturbing, since it substantially increases the likelihood that the two will meet in a common host such as a human or a pig. If this occurs, and a genetic reassortment takes place, then we could find ourselves facing a BRAND NEW hybrid virus that not only has the ability to spread easily among humans, but one that could easily kill millions of people as well. We all pray this never happens, but "never" covers a lot of time.

Between 1997 and early 2006, the CDC confirmed the following instances of bird flu viruses (remember: there are more than 100 types of bird flu) infecting humans:

- Hong Kong, 1997
- United States, 2002
- Netherlands, 2003
- United States, 2003
- Thailand & Vietnam, 2004
- Turkey & Indonesia, 2006
- China & Hong Kong, 1999
- China & Hong Kong, 2003
- Hong Kong, 2003
- Canada, 2004
- Asia & Europe, 2005
- Iraq & Nigeria, 2006

As you can see, avian flu outbreaks in humans are not exactly uncommon. This is why the current situation has the world's governments and public health authorities on edge, and very concerned that we may be on the verge of a bird flu pandemic.

Ready References

www.birdflubeacon.com

www.cdc.gov

www.nejm.org – November 24, 2005

Should you personally be worried?

Well, for a global influenza pandemic to occur, there are three conditions that must be met:

1. A new subtype of influenza A virus must be introduced into humans.
2. The virus must cause serious illness in humans.
3. The virus must be able to spread easily (especially through the air) from person to person.

In case you haven't yet realised it, conditions 1 and 2 are already fact. If the virus evolves to enable easy transmission between humans, the action will start very quickly and we must be prepared, if not as nations, then as individuals. Many researchers believe — as do I — that our luck isn't going to last forever, and we will very likely come to a day when bird flu begins a rapid, worldwide spread in humans.

If that day arrives — and I certainly pray it doesn't — I can only hope that you have followed my suggestions in this survival guide, and have prepared your family as best as possible for what the future might hold.

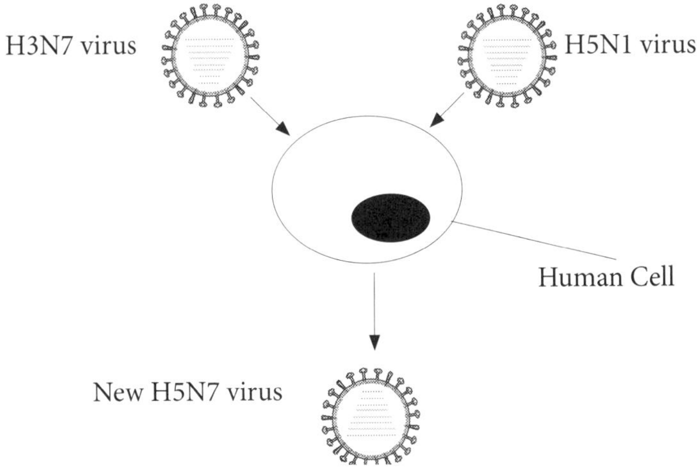

Diagram of genetic reassortment of two flu viruses in a human cell. This produces a new type of flu virus for which previous flu vaccines would be ineffective

Chapter 4: Symptoms and the Next Pandemic

"If it (bird flu) really comes and kills people as it's killing people now and it's highly transmissible, I think the statement of "the world as we know it won't exist" is true, and there's very little to be done about it." — Professor Graeme Laver

Professor Laver was a great Australian scientist and was one of the discoverers of the antiviral drug Relenza

Many of the world's leading flu experts — along with large numbers of medical doctors like me — share the belief that all of the current concern about a bird flu pandemic is definitely not misplaced. There is no way at this time to pinpoint when a pandemic might actually occur, but as long as H5N1 and similar viruses continue to circulate in both wild and domestic birds, the risk will remain.

From what we have seen in the Asian countries where the bird flu virus has infected humans, it can spread through your body with truly frightening speed, and many of its victims are young and apparently healthy. While much of the remainder of this book will focus on avoiding bird flu, along with strengthening your immune system in case you do become infected, it's also important to know the symptoms — because if you are unlucky enough to catch bird flu, **early detection may make the difference between living and dying.**

The reason that bird flu often kills, and ordinary flu is much more benign, goes back to the residual immunity most of us have for the more common flu strains. If we get sick with one of the flu viruses that make their rounds every winter, we usually have partial immunity based on a previous exposure or a flu shot. With a new flu virus like H5N1, that natural immunity is only wishful thinking and all of the symptoms we experience will be much worse.

If the H5N1 virus were to enter your body, it would head for the lungs. Then, according to Australian medical virologist Dr. Dominic Dwyer, "it promotes an immune response just like any other infection. But that's where the similarities end. Because the virus is so different to anything else our bodies have dealt with, the immune system goes into overdrive. It triggers what's called a cytokine storm, which is basically a really aggressive reaction of the immune system to the infection. The lungs fill up with fluid and cells and you can't get oxygen into your lungs and thus into your blood, and so you die."

Not a very pleasant way to go, is it, drowning from the inside? So, should you get the bird flu, knowing the specific symptoms may be critical to your survival — especially if the ordinary flu happens to be circulating at the same time, which could then result in general confusion as to what type of flu is making you ill.

Symptoms of Influenza

Bird flu:

Fever, cough, sneezing, running nose, sore throat, muscle aches (myalgia), fatigue, headache, shortness of breath and acute respiratory distress. Diarrhoea, vomiting and abdominal pain are possible. Patients can develop severe viral pneumonia, bleeding from the nose and gums, inflammation of the brain, multiple organ failure, (especially failure of the lungs and kidneys), and other severe and life threatening complications in a matter of days.

Common flu:

Fever, cough, sneezing, sore throat, sore red eyes (conjunctivitis), running nose, fatigue, headache and muscle pain. In smokers, those with other medical problems (such as asthma and chronic bronchitis) and in very old, young and immuno-compromised patients, severe pneumonia and other complications may occur.

NOTES

1. Patients with bird flu virus infections most often have lower respiratory tract symptoms such as cough and shortness of breath; whilst in the regular flu early symptoms relating to the upper respiratory tract are more common.
2. With ***any type*** of flu, there can be complications that range from dehydration to worsening of chronic conditions such as congestive heart failure, kidney failure, diabetes or asthma. In children and some adults, you may see sinus problems or ear infections.

With both bird flu and ordinary flu, patients will generally experience a high fever, with temperatures running between 38 to 40 degrees Celsius, which is 101 to 104 degrees Fahrenheit.

One very key distinguishing feature that may indicate bird flu is a shortness of breath.

In addition, it has been reported that almost all bird flu patients will have what is being called "crackles" in their chest — a sound that is easily heard by your doctor with a stethoscope placed over the bases of the lungs. Crackles are called "crepitations" by medical doctors and these signify excess fluid in the lungs.

If you feel like you have the flu, and if trouble breathing or other chest problems are among your symptoms, do not delay in seeking medical help. Your life may be on the line.

Death Rate

- **Bird flu:** Possibly in excess of 50 percent. Of the first 169 people who became infected with the H5N1 strain of bird flu, 91 of the victims — many of them young people — didn't recover.

- **Common flu**: On average, kills up to 2 percent of the people it infects, with the elderly, young children and people in developing countries most at risk. Mortality rates in developed countries are usually much lower. In a normal year, the common flu virus manages to kill up to one million people worldwide.

Are there accurate tests to see if you have bird flu?

There are diagnostic tests that can be performed in your doctor's office or in a hospital setting that will point toward ordinary flu or bird flu, as opposed to other viral and respiratory infections that may share some or many of the same symptoms. And if you think you have the flu, your doctor may recommend one or more tests. These tests are done on specimens of blood, sputum or swabs of the nose and throat. A chest X-ray should also be done.

A specialist known as a microbiologist should be contacted by your doctor, as some of the tests must be done by a specialised laboratory and instructions may be needed for special specimen handling and transport.

For more information on testing for the flu, ask your healthcare provider or go to the Web site of the Cleveland Clinic Journal of Medicine at www.ccjm.org and look for an article titled "Influenza 2005–2006: Vaccine supplies adequate, but bird flu looms" in the November 2005 issue.

Further interesting information can be found at
www.medpagetoday.com/InfectiousDisease/PublicHealth/tbl/1835

My interest in writing this book lies in helping you avoid bird flu in the first place, or if you do get it, saving you from a lethal result. All of the statistical projections I've seen indicate that a bird flu pandemic could potentially create a nightmare scenario of disease and death.

In the 1918 Spanish Flu pandemic, which was admittedly exceptional in terms of overall illness and death, the worldwide mortality rate was likely somewhere in the 2.5 percent range. Granted, we have generated huge advances in healthcare in the past 90 or so years, so it's somewhat unlikely that the death toll from any future pandemic would be nearly this high. But if that 2.5 percent figure were reached in the next pandemic, the number of deaths would be staggering. To give you some examples (and these are based on estimated population figures from July 2005), a 2.5 percent fatality rate would mean:

- Worldwide: approximately 160 million deaths
- China: approximately 32 million deaths
- India: approximately 25 million deaths
- European Union: approximately 11 million deaths
- United States: approximately 7 million deaths
- Australia: approximately 500,000 deaths

The figures listed above do represent the worst possible scenario. This data lends itself to the question: What would be the best-case scenario? A 1 percent fatality rate? This would represent 200,000 deaths in Australia and nearly 3 million deaths in the United States. What about half a percent? That's still 100,000 deaths for Australia and somewhere around 1.5 million fatalities in the Unites States. Even at one-tenth of 1 percent, 20,000 Australians and 300,000 Americans would die.

Also, you should keep in mind that deaths from a bird flu pandemic would all come in a relatively short period of time, probably 12 to 18 months. What a terrible burden that would be, not only on the families of the victims, but also on communities and society as a whole, as we tried to digest and manage the loss of so many people in such a short period of time. Are you getting a better feel for the horror that would accompany a pandemic?

Again looking back to 1918 and the Spanish Flu pandemic, it is estimated that it took this killer flu somewhere around four months to circumnavigate the globe. Today, if bird flu or any other new subtype of the influenza virus were to start spreading easily among humans, that time frame would probably be reduced to a matter of days — not even weeks, but most likely days. And the reason for that speedy spread is simple: an estimated one million people fly across international borders each day.

If, on any given day, each of the thousands of aeroplanes carrying these people only had one passenger infected with bird flu, and if that passenger was coughing or sneezing or otherwise spreading germs by touching such things as door handles, or if worse yet the infected person was a flight attendant, then the international spread of the flu virus would be well under way. Most healthy adults are thought to be able to infect others for at least a day before they know they are sick, so what might appear to be an innocent cough caused by a dry throat or a particle of dust, could in reality be a cough of death.

Stages of a Pandemic

The World Health Organization (WHO) has developed a global preparedness plan that outlines the six stages of a pandemic, which if you are interested can be found at—www.cdc.gov/flu/avian/gen-info/pandemics.htm.

To me, the most relevant — and the most frightening — aspect of international pandemics is that once one begins, the general consensus says that it will be unstoppable. It is a fact that throughout history, human intervention has **never, not once,** managed to stop a pandemic. That is an eye-opening thought, and leaves us with only two options that I can see:

- Stop the pandemic before it starts.
- Follow the advice in Bird Flu: Your Personal Survival Guide and be as prepared as you possibly can.

Can a looming pandemic actually be stopped before it gets started? This is a very good question, and the answer really depends on who is doing the talking. There are a number of pandemic prevention and preparedness efforts currently under way around the world and they could indeed have some influence on the future spread of bird flu. One focus, for instance, is on raising awareness of the dire need for early detection of the H5N1 flu in poultry. The rapid destruction of infected birds is another priority, along with seasonal flu vaccines for poultry workers and new and rigid restrictions on moving live poultry from one country to another.

An alliance of organisations led by the United Nations is working on an avian flu early warning system, which will supposedly be capable of alerting countries on the arrival of potentially infected birds. Along this same line, biothermal RFID (radio frequency identification) chips can supposedly be inserted into the breasts of poultry to alert farmers to rising temperatures in their flocks — a vital sign of the flu.

Workshops are being set up in various countries, local authorities are reportedly being trained, millions of dollars are being spent on influenza surveillance in Asia, research is ongoing to develop new H5N1 vaccines ... the list actually goes on and on. But how effective most of these measures will be is anyone's guess, especially because many of the preventive efforts are still in the planning stages.

An American epidemiologist has called a potential global bird flu pandemic "the single greatest risk to our world today." As much as I would like to disagree with this statement, I simply can't. My medical training and my research on the subject leads me to conclude that should a pandemic occur, the resulting picture will be extremely ugly. We need to prepare for a pandemic on a personal level, and by that I mean we all need to have a personal survival plan. My own survival plan is this book — and I'm more than happy to share it with you.

Ready References:

www.who.int
www.science.howstuffworks.com
www.cdc.gov

Chapter 5: Protecting Yourself from Bird Flu

"The one socially positive thing about influenza is that it's not a great respecter of person or position. You are not protected by being rich, you are not protected by being handsome or the reverse. It's a great leveller." — Dr. Shirley Fannin

To this point, we've established the potential seriousness of bird flu and looked at "why and how" it could achieve pandemic status. You understand that if bird flu is a risk anywhere in the world, then it becomes a risk everywhere — such is the flu's ability to spread. And by now you know that if a bird flu pandemic ever finds its global wings, it will most likely be left up to each of us, to a significant degree, to protect ourselves and immediate family. It's time to discuss, "How?"

How do we best protect ourself, our family or our employees? How do we evade bird flu? How do we boost our chances of surviving a pandemic?

There are never any guarantees, of course, when it comes to health or sickness or dying. And it would be an out-and-out falsehood — not to mention a violation of the medical profession's ethics — if I were to promise that I had ALL of the answers or guaranteed that you and your family could avoid and/or survive the bird flu by simply following the suggestions in this guide.

What I do pledge, though, is that my survival plan — if followed closely — will significantly reduce your chances of catching bird flu should it ever visit your neighbourhood, and significantly improve your chances of survival should you ever come down with the illness. And that's the best that anyone can offer.

NOTE: Before I go any further, I want to emphasise that the two best ways to prevent the spread of bird flu, or any other respiratory illness for that matter, are: (1) wash your hands frequently and (2) cover your mouth and your nose, preferably with a tissue, when you sneeze or cough.

If you read the newspaper or watch much TV, you will be inundated with information about antiviral drugs and vaccines and so forth and so on, but the bottom line here is you won't catch the flu if you aren't infected with the virus. And the two most common ways in which a virus is transmitted is by touching something that is contaminated and then touching your mouth, nose or eyes, or by breathing in viral germs that are suspended in the air after someone who is already sick coughs or sneezes. Nothing beats old-fashioned hygiene when it comes to preventing the flu — bird or otherwise. **This is very important to remember.**

Meanwhile, as governments and public health agencies worldwide are making elaborate and complicated plans to prevent a bird flu pandemic, I believe that aside from hand washing and covering up when you sneeze, many of the other most effective preventive measures are also among the simplest... beginning with building up your immune system. I will get into this subject in much more depth in the following chapters, which feature a wide range of foods, herbs and supplements that are known to strengthen your natural immunity.

First, I'm going to touch on four things you must address if you want to have a healthy immune system: stress, sleep, exercise and water.

- **Stress.** It is no secret in the medical profession that stress compromises your immune system, primarily by causing your body to produce more of the hormone cortisol, which in turn hampers the ability of white blood cells to fight infections. You can manage stress with exercise, meditation, yoga, rearranging your schedule to get more rest, or a combination of these and other activities. All that's really important is to find a system or a program that works for you, and then stick with it.
- **Sleep.** Getting the proper amount of rest on a regular basis is often easier said than done, especially for those of us with families and a hectic work schedule. Still, it is very important to make the effort. If you find that your personal situation oftentimes makes it impossible to get a good seven to eight hours of sleep each night, try making the time for a brief nap — even 15 minutes can work wonders — during the day. It's a fact that a rested body is a healthier body.

- **Exercise.** It is extremely important to get your body moving — and get it moving now — if you want to have a healthy immune system. In the first place, exercise will help you shed any excess fat you might have. Excess fat reduces respiratory function and readily stores toxins that are damaging to your immune system. Exercise will also reduce stress, which we've already identified as a drain on the immune system. The beauty of exercise is that it covers any number of activities, from gardening and swimming to walking. If you can do a form of exercise that gets you outside into the fresh air and sunshine, your body will benefit greatly — your brain will de-stress and your skin will make immune-strengthening vitamin D; furthermore the extra oxygen will be good for your lungs. Just do it often.
- **Water.** Your body's cells require a lot of water to work properly, with the standard recommendation being that you drink 1.9 litres (64 ounces), each day. One of the easiest ways to do this is to drink a good-size glass of water before and after each meal. Coffee and soft drinks are not good substitutes for water, as they can rob your body of nutrients that help your immune system fight infections.

Also, don't smoke cigarettes. If you're a heavy smoker you are in a precarious position if the bird flu arrives in your neighbourhood. I strongly urge you to quit as soon as possible and to get professional help for this, if needed. Light smokers and those who smoke less than five cigarettes a day, are far less vulnerable than heavy smokers; but any cigarette you inhale is doing damage to your lungs.

***Smoking damages your respiratory tract and lung tissue in many ways*:**

- It stops the tiny microscopic hairs in the airways (trachea and bronchial tubes) from cleaning the debris and mucus from the lungs.
- It causes inflammation in the mucous membranes of the airways and the tissues of the lungs so that any extra inflammation, such as that caused by a severe flu virus, may be intolerable for you.
- It damages, thins and stiffens the fragile membranes in the lung tissue across which oxygen is absorbed.

The bird flu virus causes the lung's membranes to get severely inflamed and causes holes in them so that an outpouring of fluid occurs — you literally drown from the inside. In smokers there is already pre-existing damage that makes it much easier for a nasty flu virus to cause intolerable damage that is not survivable.

Having a healthy immune system is your first line of defence against bird flu and will put you in a good position to fight off or survive the virus. This is true regardless of whether (1) you plan to travel to an area of the world where bird flu is active, (2) you worry about getting bird flu by preparing chicken or eggs, or (3) you are concerned about bird flu coming to your own area. And you will be relieved to know that there are additional precautions you can take to dispel most fears caused by 1, 2 or 3.

Vital Information for Travelling and Dining

If you're planning a trip — business or pleasure — to a corner of the world where bird flu has been reported, the first thing you should do is educate yourself about the virus (which you are doing by reading my book) and keep a list of flu symptoms (see page 37) with your travel documents. It's hard to fight an enemy you can't recognise. Next, make sure you are up-to-date on all of your vaccinations and sign up for health insurance that will cover medical evacuation if you get sick and are unable to fly home on a commercial airliner. It's also wise to carry the contact information for your country's embassies and consular offices in the places you'll be visiting, in case emergency assistance is needed.

When travelling abroad, I always take along a health kit containing basic first aid and medical supplies — including a thermometer and an alcohol-based hand rub for hand hygiene. (Don't for a moment forget the importance of keeping your hands clean!) When you arrive at your destination, it goes without saying — though I'll say it anyway — that you should avoid poultry farms and bird markets where live poultry are kept, and avoid all contact with sick or dead birds or uncooked poultry.

Is it safe to eat poultry and eggs?

Many people are concerned about the safety of eating poultry and eggs, and it doesn't seem to matter if we're talking about a restaurant or their own household kitchen. "Is it safe?" is a question I'm frequently asked. My answer is always the same, "Yes, as long as you use common sense and take a few simple precautions." The following guidelines apply to everyone equally, whether you are a veteran international traveller or someone who never ventures farther from home than the corner store. If you enjoy eating poultry and/or eggs, then you should know to:

- Purchase poultry and poultry products only from restaurants and shops that carry some sort of certification for cleanliness or obviously believe in the importance of good hygiene.
- Avoid buying or eating eggs with cracked shells.
- Wash egg shells in soapy water before handling and cooking, and wash your hands afterwards. This will remove bird faeces from the egg shells.
- Freeze, refrigerate or cook poultry as soon as possible after buying it, since any viruses that may be present will multiply rapidly at room temperature.
- Keep poultry in a container on the bottom shelf of the refrigerator to prevent drippings from falling on and contaminating other food.
- Avoid thawing frozen poultry at room temperature, which encourages any existing viruses to multiply. Instead, thaw it in the refrigerator, in or above a pan to catch the drips.
- Avoid touching the mouth, nose and eyes when handling food — particularly poultry and meat — and wash your hands for 20 to 30 seconds with soap and hot water after handling raw meat.
- Use separate chopping boards for cooked and raw poultry and do not place cooked meat back on the same surface it was on before it was cooked.
- Scrub and sanitise utensils and chopping boards with hot, soapy water and wash sponges and kitchen towels frequently with a 10 percent bleach solution or antiseptic soap.
- Cook eggs until the yolks and whites are firm and avoid recipes that say you should use raw or partially cooked eggs.

- Cook poultry to reach an internal temperature of 70 degrees Celsius (158 degrees Fahrenheit) for 30 minutes. It is suggested that you use a cooking thermometer to ensure the required temperature is reached. If poultry is well cooked, juices run clear and the meat near the bone is not pink. Flu viruses are destroyed by heat.
- The H5N1 bird flu virus can survive in low temperatures, so even if uncooked poultry has been refrigerated it should still be handled and prepared with all of the same precautions and care you would use in handling and preparing fresh poultry products.

Face Masks

Naturally, we all hope that bird flu never makes an appearance in our own neck of the woods, but it just wouldn't be prudent to count on this not happening. Again, that leaves only one option: Be prepared. And another way you can do this is by stocking up on face masks. Unfortunately, not all face masks are created equal.

If you recall, flu viruses are many times transmitted through exposure to the sneezing and coughing of an infected person. While you may resemble a mad scientist when you wear one, a face mask can definitely block out most viral germs and provide a lot of protection — as long as you have the right kind and it fits well. There are many different types of face masks, with the dust and surgical masks sold at many hardware stores and pharmacies being the least effective. Still, if these kinds of masks are all that are available to you, don't turn up your nose at one. Surgical and dust masks will prevent between 30 percent and 40 percent of airborne particles from being inhaled. Not great, but better than nothing.

The higher standard masks (defined by Australian standard AS/NZS1716 or the U.S. standard NIOSH N95) contain an inbuilt filter that blocks germs from passing through the mask. These filtering face piece masks are preferred when it comes to protecting you from the H5N1 virus. These are rated as N95, N99 or N100 — which means they are 95 percent, 99 percent and 99.7 percent effective at removing small particles from the air. Some masks are of the "use once and then throw away" variety, while others are reusable and come with replaceable filters. There are even masks that offer filters coated in a substance that will kill viruses on contact. For a brand-name review of some of the different types of face masks currently being marketed, check out the Web site www.survivetheflu.com. To purchase face masks, you can use an Internet search engine to find retailers in your community, or contact your local pharmacy.

What type of mask you choose, and how many you purchase, might depend on where you live. If your home is in a heavily populated high rise in the middle of a large city, I'd say you should have an ample stock of the best masks available. If, on the other hand, you live in a sparsely populated area where neighbours are few and far between, a smaller supply of a less costly mask might suit your needs. This is an individual decision, though when you make it you should keep two important facts in mind:

- No mask, no matter how expensive or high tech, is going to be 100 percent effective all of the time.
- If you do little or nothing else to prepare for a pandemic, it is a good idea to purchase a supply of face masks.

Infection Control Procedures

It is vital to understand the basics of infection control procedures in case a pandemic arrives in your community. These procedures will:

1. Give you good protection (though not 100 percent) against becoming infected with a respiratory virus like bird flu or new mutations of this virus. At the very least, they will reduce the amount of virus you will be exposed to, which should reduce the severity of an infection.
2. Reduce the spread of the disease in the community.

Personal Protective Equipment

The following equipment serves as an Infection Control Kit; thus, it offers you personal protection as well as reducing the spread of the virus.

Essential items include:

1. Face masks
2. Goggles that are large, well fitting and made of transparent plastic; these prevent the virus from entering your body via the lining (mucous membranes) of the eyes
3. Gloves, with disposable plastic gloves being the best — they do not need to be sterile
4. Gowns, which should be disposable and lightweight with long sleeves to go over your clothes
5. Wipes, which should be disposable for cleaning contaminated surfaces (you can get alcohol wipes, but they are more expensive)
6. Plenty of soap and detergent and alcohol-based hand rubs
7. Paper towels — these are preferable to tea towels or cloths that will be shared by other hands

Do not re-use these items if you have been around infected birds, persons or areas; dispose of them in a lined rubbish bin.

If a pandemic arrives, the essential items above could be life saving.

- **Correct order to put on your gear:** mask, goggles, gown, gloves.
- **Correct order to take off your gear:** gloves, goggles, gown, mask.

Remember: Respiratory infections like influenza are spread through the air and by touching contaminated surfaces.

For an excellent DVD presentation by the Australian Health Department on infection control, visit:
http://www.health.gov.au/internet/wcms/publishing.nsf/Content/phd-pandemic-prepared-protected.htm
I highly recommend this DVD to all people concerned about reducing their risk to all infections.

Other Safety Tips

- As much as is practical or possible, limit your exposure to people who are sick.
- If you get sick, stay home from work or school so as not to infect anyone else.
- If anyone in your house is sick, regularly disinfect doorknobs and kitchen and bathroom areas.
- Keep plenty of tissues and paper towels on hand and line rubbish bins with plastic bags and change those bags daily.
- If you are sick, avoid dairy products and foods made with wheat, as they can cause extra mucus.
- Wash your hands … wash your hands … and then wash your hands again. (Sorry, but this deserves repeating.)

Finally, it is worth noting once more that should a pandemic occur, there will likely be a lot of social unrest and many of the services that we depend on, such as food deliveries to grocery stores, will be interrupted. At the very first sign of a widespread bird flu outbreak, stock up on canned goods, bottled water and all prescription and over-the-counter medications you and your family might need.

See page 120 for the list of things you need to stockpile to survive a pandemic.

I cannot stress enough that if bird flu ever invades your part of the world, your survival may very possibly be related to how well you have prepared. And while that sounds terribly dire, I will be doing you no favour by pulling my punches. Fact is fact, and the fact here is that much about bird flu and pandemics is very distressing. But even so, the following chapters should lighten the mood a bit, as they'll show you how to strengthen your immune system through nutritional medicine.

Ready References:

- www.survivetheflu.com
- www.efsa.eu.int
- www.afic.org
- www.cdc.gov/flu

Chapter 6: Fighting the Flu with Nutritional Medicine

It is important to understand that your nutritional status greatly influences how your immune system will cope with any severe infection, such as bird flu. If you are deficient in important nutrients, the severity of an infection will be greater, and carry a higher risk of serious and potentially life-threatening complications.

If and when bird flu strikes, your body will not have any antibodies against it. To survive, especially if an effective vaccine has not been developed, you will have to rely on the proper function of your basic immune system and respiratory tract (a target area of a bird flu infection). A well-planned nutritional program will take several weeks to several months to get your immune system ready to protect you. The time required depends upon your current nutritional status, your age and co-existing diseases. Such a program will also:

- Support the health of your lungs
- Optimise the function of your immune system
- Increase your body's supply of interferon
- Make it harder for the virus to penetrate your cells
- Reduce the ability of the virus to replicate itself
- Possibly save your life

What are the most important nutrients for a strong and robust immune system?

Selenium

Selenium is a mineral that boosts all aspects of immune function, particularly by reducing susceptibility to infection. There is a widespread deficiency of selenium in the soils in many parts of the world, including Australia, New Zealand and China. Every year, it seems, new strains of the avian influenza virus evolve in the selenium-deficient areas of China — an ideal breeding ground for transmission of viruses from animals (such as poultry and pigs) to humans. These viruses spread and can easily make their way to other parts of the world.

I call selenium "**the viral birth control pill**" to describe just how important it is in helping us fight viral infections. A normally harmless or low-pathogenic virus can become far more destructive (virulent) in a person who is selenium deficient. Selenium-deficient mice infected with a mild strain (low pathogenic strain) of influenza virus developed much more severe and protracted inflammation of their lungs, compared to selenium-plentiful mice infected with the same virus. This is important since the H5N1 bird flu virus attacks the lungs in humans.

Selenium acts on the genetic material at the centre of the virus (its RNA) and this has two highly valuable effects:

1. Inhibits its ability to multiply
2. Reduces its ability to mutate into a more aggressive (virulent) form

I would strongly advise you to start taking a regular supplement of the organic form of selenium (known as selenomethionine) in a dose of 100 mcg daily. You must be regular with this, as it takes time to overcome a deficiency. Many children are deficient in selenium and require a supplement of 10 to 50 mcg daily depending on their age and weight. This would improve their immune system in leaps and bounds. In some countries, Australia included, there is a warning on the labels of selenium supplements that states they are not suitable for children under the age of 15. I find this very disappointing as there is no evidence that the correct dose of selenium is dangerous or toxic in children!

The selenium content of the soils in which foods grow will affect the selenium content of the foods. And although fish caught in their natural habitats are high in selenium, many of the fish sold for human consumption are raised in fish farms and fed pellets. For these reasons, it is not wise to rely on diet alone for your intake of selenium. Some people worry about selenium being toxic, but my research and clinical experience shows you would have to take more than 850 mcg daily (8.5 times the adult dose I recommend), on a long-term basis for this to occur. The symptoms of selenium toxicity include brittleness of the hair and nails, digestive upset, skin rashes, fatigue and nervous system abnormalities. The Food and Nutrition Board (FNB) recently set the tolerable upper level for selenium at 400mcg daily in adults. References see page 133.

For more information call Dr Cabot's Health Advisory Service and speak to a naturopath.

Australia - 02 4655 8855. USA - 623 334 3232

Zinc

It is well recognised that the mineral zinc is essential for a healthy and strong immune system. You do not want to be zinc deficient if bird flu arrives in your neighbourhood. Zinc has proven antiviral effects, and my own clinical experience and the research I've seen have convinced me that zinc can help to reduce the chances of bird flu or any influenza causing severe pneumonia. It's the pneumonia that causes bird flu victims to develop respiratory failure.

The immune-strengthening effects of zinc include:

- Protection of cell membranes from cell-damaging chemicals and viruses.
- Closure of pores in the lung's tiny blood vessels (they are called capillary membranes) to reduce trans-capillary leakage of fluid. In simple terms, zinc can help stop the lungs from filling up with fluid when inflammation occurs.
- Hardening capillaries in the lungs to reduce inflammation.
- Reducing mucous production and other respiratory secretions.
- Stimulating production of interferon (an antiviral protein produced by immune cells).

In the event of a bird flu pandemic you may need to boost your levels of zinc in a hurry, especially if you have not been taking a regular zinc supplement or your diet has been poor. Talk to your doctor about this. Supplements are available which combine zinc with selenium and vitamins E and C, thus providing a complete antioxidant. A suitable dose of zinc on a regular basis is 5 mg to 10 mg of elemental zinc daily.

To boost zinc levels quickly, use zinc lozenges. The most common types of zinc in lozenges are zinc gluconate and zinc acetate — and both inhibit viruses in the nose and throat.
Lozenge dose: 15 mg to 20 mg of zinc (as zinc gluconate or zinc acetate) every two hours, starting when you first notice symptoms and continuing until symptoms disappear. But do not take high doses like this for more than two weeks. Suitable forms of zinc as lozenges are: gluconate, acetate, chloride, sulphate, oxide, stearate or borate. No evidence of toxicity from zinc lozenges exists, though occasionally mild irritation of the mouth may occur. Don't buy lozenges that contain citric acid or tartaric acid, as these acids may block zinc's antiviral action.

Vitamin C

The importance of vitamin C to human health was enshrined by the work of two-time Nobel laureate Linus Pauling. Many other great researchers have also proved the life-saving properties of this powerful antioxidant vitamin. It seems surprising that today there are so many people deficient in vitamin C, when it is so widely available in supplement form.

One of the world's leading experts on vitamin C, Dr Thomas Levy, provides compelling evidence for its healing power in his book *Vitamin C, Infectious Diseases and Toxins: Curing the Incurable*. Dr Levy has found that vitamin C exerts a killing effect against all viruses provided enough vitamin C reaches the virus, especially in acute infections. Dr Robert Cathcart has treated thousands of severe cases of infectious diseases (including influenza) with high-dose vitamin C, and believes that very large doses of vitamin C would be required to treat a human infection with bird flu. I tend to agree with Dr. Cathcart. Unusually high doses may be administered orally as ascorbic acid or intravenously as sodium ascorbate.

Vitamin C helps fight viruses by inhibiting the protein neuraminidase, which is produced by viruses and is needed for them to grow and duplicate themselves. It also:

- Increases the killing power of your body's own immune cells
- Increases the body's production of immune-fighting chemicals such

as interferon and nitric oxide

- Increases the immune cell production of antibodies that inactivate viruses
- Reduces the inflammatory response caused by a virus in the host's tissues

All these actions of vitamin C would be very useful if you ever found yourself fighting the H5N1 bird flu virus and the life-threatening complications it can cause. While there have been no controlled vitamin C trials in humans infected by the influenza virus — perhaps because there is no money in a natural substance like vitamin C that cannot be patented — we do have good evidence that vitamin C reduces the severity of colds and flu. Indeed, results from more than 20 controlled studies of vitamin C and the common cold have been published, and they show that doses of at least 1 gram (1,000 mg) daily are able to reduce the severity and duration of colds. A recent human trial in students with viral infections of the respiratory tract found that hourly doses of 1,000 mg of vitamin C for the first six hours, with the same dose then given three times daily, reduced symptoms by 85 percent compared to a control group. If you were to come down with the bird flu virus, or any severe viral infection, this could mean the difference between life and death.

Dr. Mark Levine of the United States' National Institutes of Health agrees that vitamin C would be helpful against bird flu — if the patient takes high doses. He found that 3 grams of vitamin C, taken by mouth six times daily, produces the vitamin C blood levels necessary to exert a powerful antiviral effect. And Dr. Levine says that daily intravenous infusions of much higher doses (around 100 grams) would provide a sufficient amount of vitamin C to ensure that no virus could survive for long in your body. However, it must be pointed out that since we don't have any experience treating bird flu in humans with large doses of vitamin C, the best dose to use if you become infected is still a matter of theory.

A suggested program for vitamin C supplementation in someone with an acute influenza infection would be:

- Start with 1 gram every hour taken orally
- If this causes diarrhoea or abdominal cramping, halve the dose to 500 mg hourly
- If you don't get diarrhoea or cramping, you can take 2 grams hourly — but make sure you drink two glasses of water every hour

Some people find the ascorbic acid form of vitamin C is too acidic and upsets their stomach and bowels. If this occurs, you will probably find that the ascorbate or ester forms of vitamin C are better tolerated.

Preventative use of Vitamin C

I also suggest that you start taking 1,000 mg of vitamin C twice daily as a preventative and to keep your immune system strong. Keep a stockpile at home in a cool place and in a tightly sealed container so that you have it handy if a pandemic breaks out. Then, if that occurs, double the dose to 4 grams daily (take 1,000 mg every six hours). If you did not get any relief with this amount of vitamin C, it would be good to know a doctor who can administer vitamin C intravenously. Of course, if a severe pandemic breaks out, these types of holistic doctors may be impossible to get into see, thus it's wise to have your own stockpile of vitamin C at home.

Is there any danger in taking large doses of vitamin C?

In patients with severe kidney disease (renal failure), liver failure or cardiac failure, doses of vitamin C and the quantities of fluid with which it is administered need to be controlled strictly by a doctor. If you have a history of kidney stones, you would need to ensure that you drink plenty of water whilst taking high doses of vitamin C.

Ready References: www.coldcure.com/html/hand_2.html

Table of immune-boosting nutrients in foods

Nutrient	Food sources	Immune benefit
Vitamin C	Citrus fruits, blackcurrants, capsicums (bell peppers), kiwi fruit, guava fruit, all types of berries, tomatoes.	Antiviral effect. Increases action of immune cells (such as natural killer cells & phagocytes). Increases T lymphocytes.
Zinc	Whole grain cereals, seafood, red meat.	Antiviral effect. Reduces fluid leakage in the tissues and lungs.
Selenium	Brazil nuts, mushrooms, mussels, tuna, haddock, sunflower seeds, kidneys.	Antiviral effect. Reduces viral replication. Increases immune cells (phagocytes & T cells). Immune strengthening. Reduces many types of cancer.
Vitamin E	Nuts, especially hazelnuts and almonds, wheat germ, wheat germ oil, avocado pears, sunflower seeds, sweet potatoes—note these foods must be very fresh and kept at cool temperatures in airtight containers or the vitamin E will be destroyed.	Protects membranes of the immune cells. Increases population of immune cells (esp T lymphocytes). Increases virus fighting chemicals such as interferon. Reduces oxidative stress in the lungs caused by flu virus.
Vitamin D	Sunshine, oily fish, fish oil, cod liver oil, eggs.	Strengthens the lungs. Anti-inflammatory.
Beta-carotene-is a pre-cursor to vitamin A	All yellow and orange coloured fruits and vegetables, dark green leafy vegetables.	Anti-inflammatory. Protects cell membranes.

Chapter 7: Antiviral Foods and Recipes

All plants contain antiviral compounds, but they have not been fully tested to confirm which viruses they kill. There is, however, laboratory evidence that indicates many foods block or kill viruses — in addition to providing the essential nutrients needed for a strong immune system. Historical usage also counts; for instance, lemon has long been a cold and flu remedy.

Overall, my studies point to the fact that a diet rich in various types of plant foods is basically an anti-flu diet. All the foods covered in this chapter have been identified as containing antiviral compounds, many have been shown to improve immune functioning, and others are traditional flu remedies.

If you want to avoid a severe case of influenza, use the foods recommended here on a regular basis.

Some of my recommended foods, notably medicinal mushrooms and sea vegetables (seaweeds), are an acquired taste and I hope you will gradually get to enjoy them. If a particular food does not agree with you, or if you simply don't like the taste, you can either try it prepared in a different way, have smaller quantities mixed in with the foods you do like, or avoid it altogether because there is a wide variety of food with antiviral activity.

I have endeavoured to list these foods in order of "immune importance," but I have also considered the overall health value of the food. I am convinced that eating a wide range of the foods listed in this chapter — in as natural a state as possible — will help to reduce the severity of any influenza virus, including the feared H5N1 bird flu, and speed recovery. It is important to note that I am not recommending that eating only one antiviral food each day will either prevent or help treat the flu, so don't pick just one food you like and eat enormous quantities. A well-balanced diet is always the best diet.

Any list of antiviral foods would have to include:

- Medicinal mushrooms
- Sea vegetables (seaweeds)
- Citrus fruits, especially lemons
- The cabbage family
- The carrot family
- The onion family: onions, garlic, leeks, shallots
- Coconut flesh, full cream coconut milk and virgin cold pressed coconut oil
- Tomatoes
- Whey
- Blackcurrants and their juice
- Tea
- Walnuts
- Pomegranates
- Flavonoid-rich foods, such as citrus fruits and buckwheat
- Lignan-rich foods, such as whole ground flaxseeds
- Highly coloured fruits and vegetables, which are high in antioxidants and are much more powerful if they are fresh and in season and have been ripened naturally

Medicinal Mushrooms

A number of medicinal mushrooms are now sold as extracts, tablets or powdered remedies, and if you use these be guided by the label dosages because they come in varying concentrations. I prefer to use these mushrooms as foods. I focus on **shitake** and **reishi** mushrooms because they are well researched. They are sometimes available fresh, but you will find dried products in supermarkets, health food stores and Asian shops.

Immune strengthening effects of mushrooms

Experimentally, a compound in shitake mushrooms (lentinan) gave complete protection against a virulent influenza virus. In Japan, shitake is classed as a general tonic and used medicinally for all diseases involving low immune function. Shitake boosts immune cell function and has antiviral activity. The reishi mushroom is a longevity remedy and has a wide-ranging and beneficial immune activity.

NOTE: Other medicinal mushrooms include maitake and cordyceps, but in many countries these are usually available only in supplement combinations. The recommended amount of cordyceps is 3 to 4.5 grams twice daily as capsules or simmered for 15 minutes in water for tea.

How to use dried medicinal mushrooms

These dried medicinal mushrooms are leathery, so you need to soak them in tepid water for about 20 minutes and then slice them finely with kitchen scissors to add to rice, casseroles, stews, soups and stir-fries. For flu prevention, use at least one serving weekly. Use two to three servings a week if the flu is spreading around your neighbourhood. If you develop symptoms of the flu, take up to 15 grams daily.

Anti-flu mushroom soup recipe

8 whole dried shitake or reishi mushrooms
6 cups water
1 cup whole rice
2 carrots, sliced into pieces
3 teaspoons miso
1 tablespoon finely chopped fresh coriander and/or parsley

Soak the mushrooms in one cup water. Bring the rice to the boil in 5 cups water, and simmer for 20 minutes (less cooking time if you use other types of rice). Cut each mushroom into three or more slices, and add to the rice, together with the soaking water; simmer for further 20 minutes. Add the carrots, and simmer for a further 5 minutes. Turn off the heat, and stir in the miso and coriander. If you like ginger, add in about 2 to 3 teaspoons fresh grated root. Serve with finely cut fresh parsley and/or chives. Serves 3.

Sea Vegetables (Seaweeds)

Seaweeds are definitely an acquired taste so use very small quantities with other flavoursome foods for your first efforts. They are sold dried in packets and soften and swell once they are moistened.

Immune strengthening effects of seaweeds

Research in various countries is mainly on particular compounds in seaweed, such as fucoidans, that are active experimentally against enveloped viruses — the broad category into which influenza viruses belong.

How to use seaweeds

I suggest about two servings a week of seaweeds. Below are a few easy ways of using the types of seaweeds that you can buy in supermarkets, health food stores and Asian shops:

- **Arame and Hijiki (Hijikia).** These are good for beginners! They are relatively mild tasting and usually sold in tiny dried strips. Start with about 2 to 3 teaspoons or even less per person. You can break the seaweed into small pieces with your fingers and add to soups or casseroles towards the end of the cooking time. Another option is to break the seaweed into small pieces, moisten with a salad dressing and add to a mixed salad.
- **Nori.** This is sold in the form of paper-like sheets and is best known for its use in sushi dishes. You can also cut it into small pieces with kitchen scissors and add to rice or any moist food.

Nori strips with salmon and rice

1 fillet wild Atlantic salmon (other fish could be used but try to avoid farmed fish)
1 tablespoon soy sauce
4 sheets nori cut into segments about 5cm (2 inches) x 20cm (8 inches)
1 cup hot or cold cooked rice
1 large handful fresh herbs — optional
Juice of one lemon

Place the salmon in a small baking dish, sprinkle with the lemon juice and soy sauce. Cover the salmon with fresh herbs; then cover with foil or a lid. Bake for 30 minutes at 180 degrees Celsius (356 degrees Fahrenheit).

Carefully remove bones, in any, and flake the fish with a fork into a small serving bowl. Each person makes his or her own sushi by placing about 2-3 teaspoons of the mix at one end of a nori strip and rolling it up with the fingers. Serves two as an entrée

Nori is quite chewy if made and eaten immediately. At Asian stores you can buy special bamboo rollers to make sushi, which is then cut into bite-sized pieces ready to eat. Traditionally prepared soy sauces, such as Tamari, are healthy so read the labels before buying.

Kombu, wakame and dulse seaweeds - These are often sold in coarse strips and may be cut finely with kitchen scissors to add to cooked dishes such as stir-fries, soups, stews or casseroles.

Lemon

Lemon and other citrus fruits contain at least 15 different antiviral compounds and should be consumed daily by those serious about avoiding a nasty influenza infection, especially bird flu. Freshly squeezed lemon juice is the best source of antiviral substances and vitamin C. I drink lemon juice every day to control sinus infections and strengthen my immune system.

Fresh lemon juice as a flu preventive - *Juice of one to two lemons in warm or cold water first thing each day — you may sweeten it with a little honey or stevia. Use three parts water to one part lemon juice. You may also use two teaspoons of lemon juice per person in a salad or over steamed vegetables.*

Raw vegetables and lemon juice as an anti-flu snack

Slice finely or grate:

- 1 carrot
- 1 stick of celery
- 1 red capsicum
- ¼ beetroot
- 1 zucchini
- 1 small red radish
- 1 apple
- ¼ red onion

Other suitable vegetables to grate are - fennel root, kohlrabi & sliced fresh mushrooms.

Mix the vegetables with 4 teaspoons lemon juice mixed with cold pressed olive or coconut oil — this keeps the veggies fresh.

Keep in fridge and use as a snack throughout the day.

Lemon as a flu treatment

Put a whole lemon in a hot oven; when it starts to split, remove it and spoon out the juice. At the first sign of a sore throat, sip one tablespoon undiluted lemon juice. Please sip very small amounts at a time because it is extremely strong and you will notice the effect! If the juice is too strong for you, dilute it in warm water and honey — but because the combination of acid and sugar is not good for your teeth, give them a thorough brush immediately afterwards.

Other ways of getting antiviral properties from citrus:

- Add grated lemon peel to salads, soups and casseroles, and to baked goods such as cakes and muffins.
- Eat or juice four different citrus fruits (lemon, orange, lime, mandarin or grapefruit) daily as a preventive.
- Have one glass of citrus juice three times daily if you have the flu — use a combination of oranges, limes and lemons. If you pass the fruit through a juice extracting machine you leave a lot of the white pith attached, which makes the healing properties stronger.

The Cabbage Family

Vegetables in this family have antiviral effects that are probably attributable to their high content of the infection-fighting mineral sulphur. These foods are also excellent for the liver, which is a great protector of the immune system. If your liver is healthy, then your immune system is far less likely to become overwhelmed.

The cabbage family of foods includes broccoli, Brussels sprouts, cabbage, cauliflower, collards, kale, kohlrabi, mustard greens, radishes, turnips, swedes, rocket and watercress. I grow collards, kale and mustard greens and use the young leaves in salads, and use the mature leaves chopped finely in casseroles and stir-fries. I suggest having one vegetable from this plant family every day to keep your immune system finely tuned. Below are some tips for making these foods more popular with your family:

- Broccoli, Brussels sprouts and cauliflower need cooking until soft; otherwise, they may cause intestinal cramps and bloating. If you add about one teaspoon (for four people) of caraway or cardamom powder during cooking this will improve the flavour and help digestion.

- During cooking, add a bunch of fresh herbs that are tied together — this is called a "bouquet garni" and I generally use whatever is growing vigorously, such as oregano, thyme, sage and rosemary. These fresh herbs have antiviral properties to augment the infection fighting ability of the cabbage family vegetables. The herbal flavour penetrates the vegetables. When cooking is done, remove the herbs. If you don't have fresh herbs, use one teaspoon of dried mixed herbs or a vegetable stock cube.
- After cooking and straining the vegetables, add about one teaspoon of virgin cold pressed coconut oil per person together with a teaspoon of soy sauce or tamari. Shake the saucepan so that the additives are mixed through.
- Cabbage is more digestible in a salad if it is finely sliced or grated; sprinkle with a little apple cider vinegar and let stand for an hour before eating. Add in at least a handful of finely chopped fresh herbs, such as mint, basil, chives and parsley.
- Kohlrabi adds "body" to a green salad.
- Swedes are quite pleasant peeled, sliced finely or grated, sprinkled with lemon and cold pressed oil (coconut or olive oil) and used as a snack.
- Radish and rocket add zest to salads and strengthen the liver.

Baked cabbage

2 cups bite-sized cabbage segments
2 teaspoons olive oil
1 onion, very finely chopped (or shallots)
1 cup chopped tomato (or grated carrot)
2 tblsps fresh chives or basil, finely chopped (or 1 tsp dried herbs)
1 cup coconut cream (or soy milk)
2 eggs
2 - 4 tblsps grated soy or dairy cheese
1 tblsp soy sauce

Grease a small baking dish with the olive oil. Combine all the ingredients (except the milk, eggs and cheese) and place in the baking dish. Lightly beat the eggs into the milk and pour this over the vegetables. Sprinkle the cheese on top. Bake at 180 degrees Celsius (356 degrees Fahrenheit) for about 30 minutes. Serves 2.

The Carrot Family

Carrots contain 16 different antiviral compounds and it is probable that other vegetables in the same family (Asteraceae family) have at least some antiviral potential, including celery, fennel root, celeriac and parsnips. Grated carrots combine well in a cold salad with grated celeriac root and Italian parsley. Fennel root is a great snack food, and the tougher outer portion may be kept for use in soups and casseroles (with the stringy bits removed). One of the old-time favourites is cooked carrot and parsnips mashed together with a little tasty cheese, but to get more anti-flu action use coconut cream instead of cheese.

The Onion Family

Onions, chives, leeks, shallots and garlic are in this family (garlic is covered in detail in the chapter on culinary herbs). Onions are the best food source of the flavonoid quercetin, which has scientific support as an anti-inflammatory and antiviral compound. If you want to avoid infections use onions, garlic, leeks or chives on a daily basis. I prefer cooked onions because they are easier to digest; however, red onions (also known as Spanish onions) are delicious finely chopped in salads. Raw onions are superior therapeutically, but sometimes you have to weigh the advantages and disadvantages of eating them raw.

Liquid onion remedy for coughs and colds

2 medium onions (red or white)
3 tablespoons honey (choose good quality like Manuka honey)

Peel and finely chop the onions. Put the onions into a jar, add the honey, and stir. Leave to stand, with the lid on, for at least two hours. Label and date; use within two weeks. Take 2 to 3 teaspoons, 3- 4 times daily.

Coconut

Coconut oil contains fats (known as medium chain triglycerides) that are quickly absorbed and used for energy rather than being stored as body fat. Generally, I recommend an intake of about three tablespoons of coconut oil per week, although it's fine to have more as it's great to use for cooking. If you really like coconut, a few servings each week or a treat containing coconut full fat milk or cream can also be included.

Immune benefits of coconut - About 50 per cent of coconut oil is lauric acid, which the body converts into monolaurin. Laboratory studies show that monolaurin inactivates some bacteria and viruses, including the influenza virus. Coconut also contains fatty acids beneficial for immune function. Coconut is free of cholesterol and is a healthy, energy-boosting fat that will not increase cardiovascular disease.

For more information on the health benefits of coconut visit
www.coconutresearchcenter.org
www.kokonutpacific.com.au

How to use coconut - The therapeutic components in coconut oil are degraded if the oil is heated to the extent that it turns brown. Make sure you choose a good brand of organic virgin unrefined cold pressed coconut oil such as the **Niulife** brand available in health food stores. **NOTE**: Lite coconut milk and processed coconut oils are not likely to provide much immune benefit. So choose the full fat varieties of coconut cream and milk and cold pressed organic virgin coconut oil.

Coconut rice dessert

When cooking rice, near the end of cooking time, stir in two teaspoons per person of cold pressed virgin coconut oil. This is tastier with jasmine or basmati rice. Another option is to cook the rice in coconut milk or coconut cream. When cooked, add fresh sliced bananas, berries or mango.

Coconut and vegetables

Some Pacific islanders pour concentrated coconut cream over vegetables. Creaming fresh coconut milk is laborious, so I buy it canned and simmer it gently to get the required thickness. Another option is to add a little coconut oil to the vegetables at the end of the cooking time and the oil will drizzle through.

More fun ways of using coconuts

I sometimes buy a whole coconut (with the outer husk removed), break it into pieces with a hammer, store in the fridge and use pieces of the white "meat" as chewy snacks. Coconut cream (found in a can) is great for making smoothies with fresh fruit, water, ice and whey protein powder — mix all in a blender and drink. Yum!

Whey Powder

Whey is basically the by-product of cheese making and is very high in protein. Scientists have listed 26 biologically active compounds derived from whey that may help keep the immune system in a well-maintained state.

Immune benefits

Lactoferrin is a whey compound that seems to enhance the body's ability to fight viral infections. Animal experiments show that lactoferrin prevents infections and increases natural killer cell activity in the spleen.

How to use whey

There are two basic types of whey products:

- **Sweet whey powder** - contains milk proteins, lactose, calcium and other nutrients. It is not suitable for people with lactose intolerance or dairy allergies. It is pleasant tasting and may be used in baked goods or added to smoothies and cereals.
- **Whey protein -** there are many types of whey protein products on the market. Some contain a little lactose, others have various additives, a few are pure protein but without casein (a common allergen), and a few are branched chain amino acids only. You need to study the labels. Whey protein is not suitable for cooking and most product labels provide dosage and the preferred method of taking. Pure whey protein is not very palatable and I prefer to mix it into a soft food like yoghurt or a cooked apple. To avoid upsetting the digestive system, start with less than the label dose and take about three weeks to build up to the full dose.

Yoghurt

Probiotics are friendly bacteria found in yoghurt that keep unhealthy germs in your intestines at a low level — which is very desirable! Yoghurt has a preventive effect against infections. The yoghurt you choose must contain live cultures of friendly bacteria such as lactobacillus and acidophilus; so check labels and buy those with the highest cultures. Don't buy flavoured yoghurts containing sugar; instead, it's much healthier to add fresh fruit to plain acidophilus yoghurt.

I am not the only doctor to think that friendly bacteria found in yoghurt offer another weapon to flight the H5N1 virus. One of Australia's leading immunologists, Professor Ron Penny, is heading a clinical trial to study the bacteria called lactobacillus fermentum, which is found in yoghurt; it appears that these bacteria may be able to make the flu vaccine up to 12 times more effective. If initial trials with the regular influenza vaccine are successful, the bacteria will then be tested with a vaccine against the H5N1 bird flu virus. If the outcome is positive, the world's ability to produce adequate amounts of flu vaccine would be much improved.

Blackcurrant

Pure blackcurrant juice (especially freshly squeezed or juiced) is a rich source of vitamin C. Blackcurrant is known to contain 16 different antiviral compounds. Blackcurrant juice is readily available. Check that there is no added sugar and have up to one glass per day. You can add dried blackcurrants to biscuits and cakes or mix with raw nuts and seeds to use as snacks. Also, you can soak two tablespoons overnight in ½ cup of water and add to porridge or any breakfast cereal.

Tea

Common black tea contains 18 antiviral compounds and, experimentally, one of these compounds (theaflavin) can neutralise some types of viruses. Green tea also has antiviral activity. I suggest two to three cups daily. You can flavour teas with a slice of lemon and a teaspoon of honey or 1/6 teaspoon of stevia. If you're not fond of drinking teas, I suggest that you use tea like a culinary herb and add it to your herbal vinegar.

Walnuts and Other Nuts

All nuts are rich in flavonoids, and these compounds are known to have antiviral actions — so any anti-flu diet should include nuts. Walnuts have a surprisingly high concentration of antiviral compounds. Other nuts are likely to be somewhat antiviral and could be used in similar ways to walnuts.

How to use - Add walnuts and other raw nuts to your breakfast cereal, toss them into a green salad or a fruit salad, use them as snacks or add them to stir-fries.

NOTE: Nuts (and walnuts in particular) can go rancid quite quickly so you need to store them in airtight containers, preferably in the fridge. I usually buy walnuts in their shells in small quantities and put them in an airtight jar in the fridge.

Pomegranate

In Asia and parts of Europe, pomegranate fruit and seeds have been used for decades to treat infections, and a number of laboratory studies confirm that the seeds have antiviral activities. Not everyone likes the taste, but it is nice added to a fruit juice or fruit salad. Chickens are very fond of pomegranate — if you break open the ripe fruit for them. Giving domesticated birds some antiviral fruits and vegetables, plus a mineral supplement containing selenium and zinc, is another way of preventing human pandemics that originate in sick animals!

Flavonoid Rich Foods

Flavonoids are a class of water-soluble pigments that are found in many plants. A few thousand different flavonoids have so far been identified. While not labelled as essential nutrients, many of these compounds serve as antioxidants and are anti-inflammatory and immune balancing. They are found in fruits, vegetables, legumes, nuts, seeds and herbs. A number of flavonoids have been tested and show inhibitory effects against multiple viruses, with some tests showing that multiple flavonoids have more antiviral potential than a single compound — once again indicating that a varied diet rich in plant foods is a good anti-flu diet. Foods as diverse as soy, buckwheat, fruits and vegetables are recommended sources of flavonoids.

Soy

Soy is known to contain 16 different antiviral compounds, which means that it has been more thoroughly tested than most other foods. A healthy way of getting soy is to have it in fermented form, such as tofu.

Antiviral spicy tofu cubes

250 grams (8.75 ounces) firm tofu
1 tablespoon cold pressed virgin olive or coconut oil
1 tablespoon lemon juice or apple cider vinegar
1 teaspoon ginger powder
1 teaspoon turmeric, or use 4 teaspoons curry powder
½ teaspoon dried coriander
½ teaspoon dried mixed herbs
1 clove finely chopped garlic, optional

Cut the block of tofu into cubes (about 1.5 cm or 2 inches) and add the tofu to a baking dish. Sprinkle over the herbs, oil and lemon juice. Shake the dish so that the herbs are spread evenly. Bake in the over for 10 minutes at 180 degrees Celsius (356 degrees Fahrenheit). Turn over the cubes with a spoon, giving the dish another shake. Return to the oven for a few minutes.

This form of "roasting" makes the tofu flavoursome and improves the texture. You can use the tofu in stir-fries, add to rice at the end of the cooking time or add it cold to salads. For snacks, wrap it in pieces of lettuce or nori seaweed. The herbs can vary according to your taste and what you have in your pantry.

Tofu berry mouse

300 grams (10.5 ounces) silken (soft) tofu
2 cups fresh or frozen berries
3 tablespoons full fat coconut cream
2 teaspoons cold pressed virgin coconut oil
2 tablespoons concentrated pear or apple juice
2 tablespoons ground almonds

Blend ingredients together until smooth. Pour into four glass bowls.Chill before serving. Optional: Before serving sprinkle with chopped walnuts or some whole berries.

Serves 4.

Buckwheat

Buckwheat is a good source of antiviral flavonoids and is a seed, so it is a good alternative to grains.

Cold buckwheat salad

½ cup onion, finely chopped
1 cup buckwheat kernels
2 cups water
1 avocado
1 tomato, finely chopped
1 cup fresh mushrooms, finely chopped
½ cup soy or acidophilus dairy yoghurt
½ cup pumpkin seeds (pepitas)
½ cup freshly mixed herbs, finely chopped (parsley, chives, basil, rocket)
1 tablespoon soy or tamari sauce or salad dressing

Bring the water to boil in a saucepan. Add onion and simmer for five minutes. When the buckwheat has cooled, gently combine all the other ingredients, except the lettuce. Place mixture in a serving bowl. Wash and drain the lettuce leaves. Place the lettuce leaves on a separate plate. People serve themselves by putting about a tablespoon of the buckwheat salad onto a lettuce leaf and rolling it up to eat with their hands.

Serves 4-6.

Vegetarian protein loaf

2 cups water
1 finely chopped onion
2 cups buckwheat kernels
1 cup soy flakes
2 vegetable stock cubes, for flavouring
1 cup linseed meal
1 cup chopped zucchini or celery
1 cup chopped snow peas or green beans
1 cup grated raw carrot
1 cup finely chopped green herbs (chives, parsley, fennel, etc.)
1 teaspoon each of chilli, ginger and turmeric powder
4 eggs, lightly beaten
3 tablespoons sesame or caraway seeds

Place the onion and water into a large saucepan and bring to the boil and simmer a few minutes. Add the soy flakes, buckwheat, zucchini, snow peas and stock cubes, stir and let simmer for a few minutes. Turn off the heat and mix in all the other ingredients except the sesame seeds. Pour the mix into a greased baking dish with a capacity of at least 2 litres (2.12 quarts). Form the top into a loaf-like shape, sprinkle the seeds on top. Bake for about 40 minutes at 180 degrees Celsius (356 degrees Fahrenheit). Serve with a sauce of humus or cooked tomatoes, garlic and chives. The same or similar ingredients can be made into burgers, cooked in oven (not fried). Can be frozen and reheated, or used cold broken up into a salad.

Makes about 8 servings.

Lignan Rich Foods

Lignans are basically fibre-rich foods — the highest sources are whole ground linseeds (flaxseed), pumpkin seeds and berries. All whole grains contain lignans, but refined grains do not. Studies indicate that lignans can exert some worthwhile antiviral effects.

Antiviral biscuits

5 tablespoons unrefined honey
5 tablespoons tahini
1 cup whole ground linseeds
1 cup dried blackcurrants
¼ cup lemon peel
½ cup buckwheat seeds
½ cup desiccated coconut
½ cup pumpkin seeds
½ cup whey powder or substitute millet meal or oat flakes*
½ cup soy flour

*Melt the honey and tahini together in a large saucepan (don't boil). Turn off the heat and stir in the rest of the ingredients, mixing thoroughly. Tip mixture into a well-greased biscuit tray or baking dish. Flatten with your hands — as the mixture is hard to flatten, run your hands under the cold water tap as you are pressing the mix into the dish … this also moistens the biscuits. Bake at 150 degrees Celsius (302 degrees Fahrenheit) for about 20 minutes. When still slightly warm, cut into small squares. Store in fridge. If you find the biscuits too dry, use less of the dry ingredients. Makes about 30 "chewy" biscuits. *Contains lactose and is not the same as whey protein, the latter not being suitable for cooking in this way.*

Immune boosting porridge

½ cup rye, barley or oat flakes
½ cup whole ground linseeds (flaxseeds)
1 cup water
1 peeled and grated (or finely diced) apple
Handful of raisins or chopped figs
2 teaspoons poppy or caraway seeds

Place all the ingredients in a pot, bring to the boil. Simmer for a few minutes. Turn off the heat and let it stand with the lid on for 5-10 minutes. Serve with plain acidophilus yoghurt and a light sprinkle of sesame seeds. Serves 2.

To get more lignans, add raw seeds to porridges, biscuits, muffins and rissoles; use whole grains. Products such as barley flakes and rye flakes can be added to casseroles or used as thickening agents.

Carotenoids — Immune Modulators

There are various types of carotenoids (pigments) and they are found primarily in green leafy vegetables (especially collard, kale and spinach) and yellow and orange fruit and vegetables (including sweet potatoes) and red foods (such as tomatoes, red capsicum and guava). Generally green and any brightly coloured edible foods are rich in immune-strengthening substances. For instance, tomatoes contain 19 different antiviral compounds. Apart from the fact that large amounts of raw foods may be hard to digest for some people, there is evidence that important carotenoids are absorbed into your cells more effectively if they are cooked, so try to get more cooked tomato and carrot into your recipes.

Quick immune strengthening soup

1-2 peeled and chopped onions (depending on size)
5 cups peeled and chopped pumpkin*
5 cups (approx.) water
1 teaspoon mixed dried herbs or 2 tablespoons fresh herbs
1 vegetable stock cube
200 grams (7 ounces) plain acidophilus yoghurt

*Simmer the onion in water for about 5 minutes while you are chopping the pumpkin. Add the pumpkin, and sufficient water to cover the pumpkin and simmer for 10 minutes. Add the herbs and stock cube, stirring them through. Allow to cool. Put about half the vegetables in a blender, add about 100 grams (3.5 ounces) of low fat yoghurt, blending until smooth; then repeat this process with the rest of the vegetables. Reheat and serve with a dab of yoghurt and chopped chives or parsley. For lunch serve with pumpernickel bread spread with humus. Serves 4-6. *The same recipe may be used for carrots, broccoli, spinach, mushroom or tomatoes.*

Antioxidant Foods

Many of the best antiviral foods are fruit and vegetables. They contain antiviral compounds because the plants themselves need protection from viral diseases.

To increase your fruit and vegetable intake:

- Always have a piece of fresh fruit with breakfast.
- Aim to have a salad or vegetable soup with lunch and cooked vegetables plus a salad with dinner.
- Prepare veggie snacks for the day and keep them in the fridge.
- In summer, keep fruit refrigerated to use for snacks.
- Use fruit as an entrée; e.g. slices of rock melon or pineapple or orange and mandarin segments in a green salad.
- Serve lettuce leaves whole at the table and let the family put hot or cold food in them. Mignonette lettuce leaves are the right size but imperial or other types of lettuce can be broken into suitable sizes for this purpose.

Raw juices are essential for people with small appetites, nausea or digestive problems because they can provide a concentrated boost of antiviral compounds. Raw juices are also vital for people who don't eat a wide variety and quantity of raw fruit and vegetables. If you have the flu you may lose your appetite and feel too sick to take remedies or eat very much. The old adage of "feed a cold, starve a fever" is not good advice because you need nutrients and antiviral compounds to fight the flu. Raw fruit and vegetable juices will fill the gap and are usually well tolerated. If they are too strong, simply dilute them 50 percent with water or pass extra oranges, celery or apples through the juicer.

Flu preventive juice recipe

Juicing a combination of carrot, orange, lemon, apple, celery and tomato, plus a knob of garlic, makes a wonderful antiviral drink. The garlic is optional and can be replaced with a small amount of red onion or red radish.

Flu Treatment Juice Recipe

2 oranges
1 lemon
1 lime
1 clove garlic or 1 small red radish or ¼ small red onion
2 red apples

Pass the above through the juicer, then add the juice to the blender, add ½ cup fresh or frozen blackcurrants, and blend.

Antiviral stir-fry vegetables and fruit

1 onion, finely sliced
2 stalks celery, diced
1 carrot, diced
1 green capsicum, diced
1 cup chopped spinach leaves
1 handful chopped Italian parsley leaves (or other green herbs such as basil, coriander etc)
2 slices fresh pineapple, diced
½ mango, diced (optional)
2 tablespoons cold pressed virgin coconut oil (Niulife brand is excellent)
1 tablespoon honey, optional
1 red chilli diced finely, optional
1 tablespoon soy sauce
1 tablespoon lemon juice
1 tablespoon tomato paste or 1 diced fresh tomato

You can add other vegetables, tofu or seafood.

Heat the oil and gently cook the onion while you chop the celery and carrot. Add a few tablespoons of water (or leftover tea), then add the celery and carrot. Chop and add the capsicum. When cooking mixed vegetables, I always start with the ones that need the most cooking. Then add the spinach and parsley. Lastly add the fruit, honey, soy sauce, lemon juice and tomato; simmer for a few minutes. Serve with cooked rice or barley.

Serves 4.

Antiviral salad

A selection of **raw**, **grated** vegetables, such as carrot, red radish, celeriac, fennel root, kohlrabi, beetroot and cucumber, make a good antiviral salad.

Also beneficial are:

Mixed sprouts, such as alfalfa and mung beans
Salad greens, especially rocket
Finely chopped mushrooms
Mixed fresh herbs (such as parsley, chives, coriander, sweet basil, mint)
Tomato
Grated soy cheese
Pumpkin seeds

Other extras

Olives
Walnuts or cashews
Cooked, cold wild rice or chick peas or beans
Finely chopped cabbage (Prepare at least 30 minutes in advance of the meal, sprinkled with lemon juice or apple cider vinegar to help with digestion.)
Cooked, cold cauliflower or broccoli, these are hard to digest raw
Cooked, cold beans, uncooked green beans are hard to digest
Bite-size pieces of cooked, cold soy burgers or meat loaf
Hard-boiled eggs
Flakes of cold fish
Roasted savoury tofu cubes
Avocado
Wedges of peeled citrus fruits, such as oranges, mandarins or limes

The current trend of serving large green lettuce leaves as a salad is a real turn off. Try making a chewy, filling salad rather than just having green leaves. I make a salad dressing using a little tamari plus vinegar or lemon, with cold pressed olive or Niulife coconut oil, but you may enjoy something else.

Antiviral salad dressing

1 tablespoon cold pressed olive oil* or cold pressed coconut oil
2 tablespoons lemon juice or herbal or apple cider vinegar
1 tablespoon soy sauce or tamari
1 teaspoon mustard powder
1 tablespoon finely chopped fresh basil, chives, thyme, oregano or 1 teaspoon dried herbs.

Optional extras:

1 tablespoon tomato juice, 1 clove crushed garlic, pinch of hot chilli powder.

Mix the dry ingredients to a paste with the lemon juice in a glass jar. Add the oil and herbs. Put the lid on and shake until the ingredients are thoroughly mixed. Store in fridge. Serves 4.

**Some of the compounds in olive oil have antiviral effects.*

NOTE: The combination of plants in oils standing at room temperature can lead to a build up of botulinum toxin, so use these immediately or store in the fridge.

Beans

Both kidney and soybeans have tested positively for antiviral compounds, and it is likely that all legumes have some benefit to the immune system because they contain lignans and isoflavones that are known to have antiviral properties. All dried legumes (beans, chickpeas, etc.) must be soaked and thoroughly cooked; otherwise, they are not absorbed and can upset the digestive process. You can also buy them pre-cooked in cans. To ensure that beans will be well digested, I add herbs to them during cooking, including tarragon, caraway and a little chilli. Remember, culinary herbs are disease preventing and antiviral.

Chickpeas are my preferred legume. I use a pressure cooker, cook them in bulk and freeze for later use. Chickpeas are tastier if, after cooking, you dry roast them in the oven with herbs and vinegar. They may be used as a snack, mixed into cooked rice or into a cold salad.

Vinegar

Undiluted apple cider vinegar can kill a variety of micro-organisms when applied directly. Although there is no published scientific evidence that vinegar is antiviral in humans, it is at least indirectly helpful because it improves digestion and absorption; therefore, your immune cells are better nourished. Use:

- 1-2 teaspoons apple cider vinegar per person in a salad dressing
- 1 teaspoon per person over rice, cooked vegetables or any savoury food.
- 1 tablespoon rubbed over chicken or meat before cooking

Immune Strengthening Herbal Vinegar Recipe

1 bottle of apple cider vinegar (about 500 ml or 16 ounces), plus one spare empty bottle with a lid

3 - 4 teaspoons of powdered or crushed herbs, such as ginger, turmeric, mustard, thyme, caraway, coriander and/or cumin

1 - 2 bags of herbal tea, such as camomile, peppermint or lemon balm

1 handful of fresh herbs, such as sage, basil, fennel, rosemary, oregano and/or lemon balm (large leaves should be cut into smaller pieces)

You can use various culinary herbs and spices, plus add in chilli and garlic if you wish. Refer to the lists in chapter 9 on culinary herbs. You can use fewer herbs and substitute all dried herbs if you don't have any fresh. However, if you are using all dried herbs, use a maximum of about 12 teaspoons. The vinegar acts as a preservative and draws the healing components out of the herbs; it should keep for at least six months. Once the fluid is used, the herbs are "exhausted" and you need to make a new bottle.

Ten percent vinegar in water is useful as a wash for removing micro-organisms from fruits and vegetables. Don't use fruit and vegetable peels unless they're home grown. A vinegar solution will not get rid of all the dangers as in this self-serve age, many hands have touched much of our fresh food. A vinegar wash before use may prevent infections. Undiluted apple cider vinegar may be used for cleaning kitchen cutting boards and benches. The smell disappears overnight.

If you buy raw chicken, give it a thorough wash inside and out with undiluted apple cider vinegar, which will barely affect the taste and acts as a tenderiser. Make sure to wear disposable plastic gloves or wash your hands in hot soapy water straight afterwards.

I use organic chickens — which may or may not be less prone to bird flu — and stuff the inside with fresh rosemary and other culinary herbs. I cook the chicken in an oven bag with a tablespoon of herbal vinegar and at least two cups of red wine (the alcohol is evaporated in the cooking process and the wine provides antioxidant and antiviral flavonoids). In addition I add in ½ cup of buckwheat kernels (to thicken the wine and provide more flavonoids), plus some garlic, chopped onion and a little tamari. Always cook chicken really well, so that the meat falls away easily from the bone.

Vinegar side effects and cautions

People with acid reflux (heartburn) may not tolerate vinegar well, although most can handle a little on food. I do not recommend you have vinegar in water on an ***empty*** stomach because you don't need acid in an empty stomach. It's very good to sip small amounts of the water-diluted vinegar during meals. Vinegar may be therapeutic, but do not have more than three teaspoons per meal and do not give vinegar to infants.

NOTE: Apple cider vinegar is the most healthful of all the different types of vinegar. You can use other types, such as rice and balsamic, but there is no specific information about their antimicrobial properties.

In this chapter I have emphasised the importance of plant foods, but that does not mean you should avoid protein. Protein deficiency impairs your immune function and reduces the protection you get in your blood and lymph circulation. Adults need at least 45 grams (1.5 ounces) of good quality protein daily.

Good sources of protein include-

Lean lamb, organic eggs and poultry, organic beef, local fresh seafood or canned oily fish, plain acidophilus yoghurt and whey. Good quality cheese but avoid processed sliced or cream cheeses.

First class protein can also be obtained by combining legumes (chickpeas, lentils or beans) with nuts and seeds at the same meal.

Dietary fats and the immune system

Unhealthy dietary fats such as margarine, processed vegetable oils and deep fried foods which contain transfatty acids. These damaged fats reduce the ability of immune cells to kill viruses. The healthy fats recommended in this chapter, such as cold pressed olive and coconut oils, along with raw nuts and seeds, actually strengthen immune function.

You may read about the benefits of moderate alcohol intake, but everyone's idea of moderate is somewhat different. In my opinion, it's one drink for women and two drinks for men per day. Anything above this increases susceptibility to viruses and reduces immune cell function.

Changing your diet and lifestyle can be stressful, but at the very least you should try to add two healthy foods or recipes each week, drink (make or buy) raw juice several times a week, and drink the juice of two lemons every day. If you do this without delay, that's an excellent start to your personal bird flu survival plan. It is also a plan to strengthen and optimise your immune system. A strong immune system will greatly increase your chances of surviving many types of severe infections and reduce your risk of cancer.

Chapter 8: Antiviral Medicinal Herbs

The medicinal herb recommendations in this chapter are based on (1) tradition or historical use, (2) the clinical experience of professional herbalists and (3) laboratory tests and clinical trials. All plants contain literally hundreds of compounds; consequently, medicinal herbs have a number of uses. Most herbs with antiviral properties also have an antibacterial and antifungal action; this means they are also useful for preventing and treating secondary infections that follow the flu.

Within each sub-heading I have attempted to list the herbs in order of their importance to fighting the flu, but since many plants have not been fully tested, the order is not precise. Asian ginseng, for instance, is ideal for flu prevention — especially if stress is a major problem. St. John's wort might be chosen instead if you have mild to moderate depression. Nothing in your body works in isolation, and factors such as depression and stress weaken immune function. When you're faced with a potentially serious infection such as bird flu, you need to first strengthen your weakest link.

Liquid Herbs

Medicinal herbal extracts are made according to specific pharmacopoeial directions, such as fine powdering, soaking in a particular alcohol and pressing with specialised equipment. Extracts are concentrated. If you have access to an olive tree, for instance, you could simply break up olive leaves and make them into a tea (infusion), but this may not represent a medicinal dose because you don't know if the therapeutic compounds have been effectively extracted simply by immersing in water. The alcohol in herbal extracts is used to draw out the therapeutic components and it also acts as a preservative.

If you have liver problems or do not wish to have alcohol for any reason, you can remove the alcohol from herbal extracts as follows: Put 100 ml (20 teaspoons or 3.3 ounces) of liquid herbs together with 25 ml (5 teaspoons) of distilled water in a small saucepan. Gently simmer for a few minutes with the lid off. You will see the alcohol evaporate. Turn off the heat, let the remedy cool, return it to the bottle and store it in the fridge. **NOTE:** I do not recommend herbal tinctures because they contain one part herb to five parts of alcohol/water; therefore, the herbal content is too low to treat the flu.

Other Forms of Medicinal Herbs

Some herbs are available as teas but they are generally unpalatable and relatively weak because soaking in hot water does not effectively draw out all the therapeutic components. Decoctions are often used for hard plant materials, such as leathery leaves and bark. This involves boiling in water and then straining.

To make herbal teas and decoctions more palatable:

- Add one teaspoon of honey or 1/6th teaspoon of stevia per cup
- Combine with another tea that you like, such as ginger or peppermint
- Add slices of lemon, orange or lime or a little of their juice
- Allow the tea to cool and mix it 50/50 with a fruit juice
- Make into an iced tea in a long glass with crushed ice, slices of fruit, some fruit juice and peppermint leaves.

The majority of herbs mentioned in this and the following chapter are also available as tablets or capsules and, depending on the manufacturing process, can be very concentrated.

Using Medicinal Herbs

Herbs can be used singly or in formulas, with formulas tending to be more potent. In nature, all plant compounds are somewhat variable depending on the age of the plant, the soil and the climate and so on — but generally this does not have a huge impact on the therapeutic effect because the overall therapy comes from all the herb's components. Health food store or pharmacy-bought herbal products are usually standardised (this means they contain a specified level of the main therapeutic compounds).

Using a variety of herbs over a period of time should produce the most therapeutic benefits. A number of databases, Web sites and reviews give details about antiviral herbs. Ref (1) see page 133.

There are a number of herbs that provide antiviral protection in various ways, and I consider the top four to be olive leaf, ginseng, echinacea and St. John's wort.

Olive Leaf

The Health Science Institute of America says about this herb "Nature's most promising antibiotic, antiviral and antifungal agent is a compound derived from the olive leaf called calcium elenolate. As the number of drug-resistant superbugs continues to increase, so will the urgent need for olive leaf extract"

Olive leaf has a long history of use in Europe for treating infections and fevers.

Dr. J. R. Privitera provides a method of using olive leaf that was first published in the ***Pharmaceutical Journal*** in 1854: Boil a handful of olive leaves in a quart of water (1.2 litres) down to half its original volume. Then administer the liquid in the amount of a wineglass every three to four hours until the fever is cured. **NOTE:** This is a decoction and is stronger than simply making a tea from the leaves. The remedy would be more potent if the leaves were broken into small pieces. Not all herbs, however, are suitable for boiling. For example, it is the aromatic oils in peppermint and chamomile that provide important flu benefits, and these oils are evaporated by heat.

Known immune benefits of olive leaf

In the 19th century it was thought that a bitter substance in the leaves was the anti-infection ingredient, and subsequently this was found to be oleuropein. This ingredient protects the plant against many insects and micro-organisms, and is considered to be largely responsible for antiviral, antibacterial and antifungal effects. A study on mice shows that oleuropein improves immune function.

Ref (1). The leaves also contain flavonoids and tannins that lab studies confirm as useful antivirals. Ref (2).

Dr Privitera uses olive leaf extract in his clinic for a variety of infections and he considers that many people *"who lead stressful lives or who may be particularly susceptible to colds and viruses may benefit from long-term use of olive leaf extract as a preventive agent."* Ref (3). He also uses olive leaf on patients with persistent flu symptoms. Bastyr University lists olive leaves as a remedy for viral and bacterial infections, especially the flu. Ref (4).

How to use olive leaf

You can make a decoction by boiling the leaves as described above, or you can buy capsules, tablets and liquid extracts over-the-counter. For flu prevention purposes, a dose of around 1,000 mg a day is suggested and this may be taken for up to six months. For treatment of respiratory tract infections, I recommend a dose of 1,000 mg four times daily for one week. Take it with food such as fruit.

NOTE: There are no known side effects of taking olive leaf, but people with heavy loads of virus or bacteria in their bodies may experience "die-off" or detoxification symptoms such as headaches. I have not experienced this in my clinic and it is unlikely at the levels I recommend. If you suspect, however, that this is happening to you, stop taking the remedy for a few days and then restart at a very low dose.

Asian Ginseng

In addition to centuries of traditional and practitioner evidence, there are more than 3,000 published scientific papers on the health benefits of Asian ginseng. Ginseng is classed as an adaptogen, meaning that it is a natural non-toxic remedy that provides support during times of physical and mental stress. One of the primary attributes of Asian ginseng is its ability to strengthen the immune system. Ref (1).

How to use ginseng

Ginseng is available in varying strengths as teas, tablets and various types of liquid extracts. Herbalists, naturopaths, online companies, health food stores and pharmacies stock it. This herb is best taken in the morning, otherwise it may prevent sleep.

Dosage and duration of treatment

The dose range of liquid extracts is between 1 ml and 5 ml per day, depending on the potency of the ginseng. Daily dosage for tablets is usually between 400 and 2,000 mg, but products come in varying concentrations so always be guided by the label dose. If you are using tea or a decoction, I suggest one cup per day. Ginseng should not be taken for more than three months without at least a month's break. An option for flu prevention is to have a month's course and then alternate with another remedy. **NOTE:** Ginseng is not to be used during an acute infection, although it is a useful for recovery. Do not take ginseng if you are on pharmaceuticals, as there have been reports of interactions with warfarin and other prescription drugs. Not recommended during pregnancy or for children. Not suitable in hot, feverish conditions or in "manic" phases of depression.

Other forms of ginseng

- **American ginseng** is an adaptogen with similar constituents to Asian ginseng, although the proportions of the various therapeutic compounds are different. My experience is that it is not as stimulating as Asian ginseng. A scientific trial of 200 elderly people showed that 200 mg of American ginseng twice daily, starting at the beginning and taken up to the end of the flu season, resulted in fewer laboratory-confirmed influenza cases compared to a placebo. Ref (2).
- **Siberian ginseng** is also an adaptogen. My experience is that Siberian ginseng is suitable for young people and sensitive women. A human study shows that it helps the immune system in various ways, such as increasing interferon and activating immune cells. A liquid extract of Siberian ginseng specifically inhibited the replication of influenza A. Ref (4). Large-scale trials have been carried out

on Russian workers, and those who received ginseng had fewer incidences of influenza and other infections. Also, sickness was less severe in those who got the flu. Ref (5).

Echinacea

There are three different species of Echinacea — namely, Echinacea purpurea, angustifolia and pallida — and are all used therapeutically. Some products contain the whole plant, some the roots only and some the aboveground parts only. Herbalists have always maintained that the therapeutic effect comes from the *combined* action of all the constituents, and that herbs are nothing like pharmaceuticals. The fact that a number of scientific studies show immune or antiviral effects from at least five groups of different compounds in echinacea supports its long history of use.

Known immune benefits of echinacea

It has been shown repeatedly that all echinacea species stimulate phagocytosis, which basically means that invading micro-organisms are ingested and destroyed by immune cells. According to Rob McCaleb, president of the U.S. Herb Research Foundation, echinacea increases the number of immune cells in the human body and stimulates production of interferon. Ref (1). Echinacea has been subjected to 21 medical trials, most of which support it for preventing and treating symptoms of the common cold and flu. Ref (2) lists some of these trials.

How to use echinacea

Echinacea is readily available as tablets and as fluid extracts. The exact dosage depends on the type of echinacea product, as some are more concentrated than others. As a general guide, I suggest around 1,000 mg daily for two to eight weeks when used as a preventive. There is some debate, however, about the ideal duration because of suspected tolerance (the body gets used to the remedy and it is no longer effective). It might be wise to alternate echinacea with one of the other preventive remedies on a monthly basis.

Echinacea may also be used as a flu treatment, but it should be at the maximum dose for two days (3,000 to 5,000 mg daily, if tolerated) and then the label dose for a further seven days — and ideally the treatment should start at the first sign of the flu or a cold.

NOTE: Echinacea is safe and well tolerated, although the possibility of allergic reactions cannot be ruled out and it should be avoided in those with severe allergies. Asthmatics should not take it without checking with their doctor first. Reactions such as diarrhoea, rashes and wheezing occasionally occur with high doses, but these are rare. The news media recently reported that echinacea is not effective for preventing and treating the common cold. The study on which this conclusion is based was flawed. Ref (3).

St. John's Wort

Two compounds in St. John's wort (hypericin and pseudohypericin) have antiviral activity against enveloped viruses, and this broad category includes influenza viruses. Ref (1). These two compounds are flavonoids that produce a strong claret colour that can be seen in liquid extracts of St. John's wort. Various components in the herb have a wide variety of actions, including antimicrobial and antibacterial, which indicate that St John's wort is likely to prevent both the flu and secondary infections. The whole herb also produces a range of therapeutic effects and works to counteract depression and anxiety, both of which are linked to decreased immune function.

How to use St. John's wort

St. John's wort is readily available in tablets and liquid extracts, some of which are standardised. The potencies are variable so you need to follow each label's dosage instructions. Generally, St. John's wort is prescribed for periods of between one to six months.

NOTE: There have been a few reports of sensitivity to sunlight, therefore do not sunbathe or use ultraviolet treatment while taking St John's wort. The herb may decrease the effectiveness of oral contraceptives. Do not take St. John's wort without your doctor's approval if you are taking prescribed pharmaceuticals. Pregnant women should take this herb only if prescribed by a practitioner.

Astragalus

The U.S. Herb Research Foundation states that astragalus stimulates virtually every phase of immune system activity. Ref (1). Astragalus is a good tonic that could be used to ***prevent*** the flu and to help recuperate ***after*** the symptoms have passed, but European herbalists tend not to prescribe it during an acute infection. This traditional Chinese medicinal herb is available over-the-counter in Australia and many other countries as a single remedy and in tablet formulas.

Hops

Hops is a traditional sleep remedy, and getting a good night's sleep improves immune functioning. It is not prescribed to depressed people and is best taken at night. Hops contains 14 different antiviral compounds. Professional herbalists always stock hops and you will find it in some over-the-counter insomnia remedies

Celery Seed

Although not a traditional respiratory remedy, celery seed has a high concentration of antiviral compounds. Seed remedies are highly concentrated and best taken as tablets. These are readily available over-the-counter.

Medicinal Herbs for Flu Treatment

If you are unlucky and get the flu, there are many herbs that have been used successfully to reduce the severity and duration of symptoms. Generally, with acute infections such as the flu you are looking for quick results, so maximum label doses should be used if tolerated — but for one week or less. Herbs, like antiviral drugs, work much better against the flu if you start at the first sign of infection.

Three of the most important herbs used as flu remedies are:

1. Thyme

In herbal tradition, both common and wild thyme have been used primarily as cough remedies and for treating infections of various kinds. Laboratory studies show that thyme contains 19 different antiviral compounds. Various studies confirm that thyme also has antibacterial action. Thyme is especially useful because it can help offset secondary infections from opportunistic bacteria after you are weakened by the flu. Thyme helps loosen and expel mucus from the bronchial tubes and lungs and, at the same time, relaxes the chest.

In my clinical experience, thyme is a very powerful anti-flu remedy. Thyme is also a component of some cough elixirs for children that also contain olive leaf and vitamin C. You can buy thyme as a culinary herb and use about ¼ teaspoon per cup of water as a tea, or you can strain it carefully, let it cool and use as a gargle. Over-the-counter cough tablets and syrups often contain thyme, and herbalists commonly prescribe the liquid extract in a formula. A medicinal dose of thyme by itself is 1-2 grams, one to three times daily. Lesser quantities are used in formulas where it is combined with other herbs.

NOTE: The isolated essential oil of thyme is extremely powerful and not recommended for self-treatments. The liquid extract is not recommended during pregnancy, though there is no evidence of harm from small quantities used in cooking.

2. Elder

The flowers of elder have been made into various types of remedies for centuries and used to treat fever, respiratory infections and excess mucus. Elder is in the honeysuckle plant family, and Chinese honeysuckle is also a successful flu remedy. Laboratory tests support its historical use and verify that elder has antiviral activity and boosts immune function. A theory is that elder renders viruses non-functional by staining and coating them. There are good studies supporting the antiviral effects of elder in subjects with influenza.

Elder flower wine

Elder is a large shrub producing white flowers and it grows readily in most areas. Cut off a whole flowering clump. Remove the individual flowers and soak in five times their weight of white wine for two weeks in a sealed bottle. (The alcohol in the wine helps draw out the therapeutic components.) Strain and retain the liquid in small, sealed bottles for immediate or future use. Before using, gently simmer in a saucepan for a few minutes to evaporate the alcohol, and drink it hot and flavoured with a teaspoon of honey and some added mint or aniseed. This will help you sweat — and then cool you down.

Dosage and duration of treatment

Tablets containing elder and elder teas are available over the counter and some professional herbalists will stock liquid extracts. As a general guideline, the daily dosage of elder tea or tablets ranges from 2 to 5 grams.

NOTE: It is safer to use the flowers, as other parts of the plant may be toxic in very large doses. Not recommended during pregnancy and lactation

3. *Licorice*

Licorice has a long and varied history of use, including as a soothing remedy for coughs and sore throats. It is also known from laboratory evidence that a compound in licorice (glycyrrhizin) inhibits the growth of several viruses and inactivates virus particles. This compound also helps interferon production and promotes immune cell function. Ref (1).

Licorice is an ideal cough remedy because it helps loosen and expel mucus, while at the same time relaxing the lungs and bronchial tubes. The whole herb has some antiviral and antibacterial activity. Ref (2). Licorice is available over the counter as a tea and in some tablet formulations. Most herbalists prescribe liquid extracts as part of a formula. For self-treatment, the maximum dose is 2 ml of liquid extract twice daily or 3 grams of powdered herb daily. Do not take for more than a month without a two-week break.

NOTE: Do not use licorice without your doctor's advice if you are taking pharmaceuticals. Not suitable during pregnancy, or for patients with kidney disease or hypertension. Also, please be aware that licorice candy is unhealthy and is in no way connected to pure licorice root, from which herbal remedies are made.

Other Medicinal Herbs with Antiviral Activity

Pau D'arco

This herb is active against a number of viruses, including influenza. Ref (1). It contains compounds that are known to increase immune function and exert antiviral activity. Pau d'arco tea/tablets are available over the counter. Most herbalists stock the liquid extract.

Thuja

Thuja acts on both naked and enveloped viruses and therefore it is presumed to have wide antiviral activity. In this case, scientific investigation confirms and supports traditional use.

Chamomile

Chamomile contains 16 different antiviral compounds. Chamomile tea is more palatable mixed with thin slices of fresh ginger root and a little Manuka honey.

Baical Skullcap

Baical skullcap is recommended for hot, infectious conditions, such as the flu. At least 10 different research papers confirm the antiviral activity of the herb, including anti-influenza activity. Ref.(3). The only disadvantage to baical skullcap is the taste, and this can be masked by mixing it in apple juice and adding a little cinnamon. Most herbalists and Asian stores stock baical skullcap.

Herbal Combinations may work best

Recent scientific research suggests what herbalists have always known: Two or more different herbs working together will provide more useful antiviral activity than either herb working alone. It's a fact that combinations of herbs are usually complementary or synergistic. A number of herbs help prevent and treat acute upper respiratory viral illnesses such as the flu, and the best evidence for this is their long history of clinical use by practitioners.

NOTE: If you are seeing a herbalist, always insist on getting a list of everything in a formula – in case of allergic or other reactions or an exceptionally good result.

When formulas are prescribed the quantity of each individual herb is reduced. If you are self-treating and decide to take, say, two or three herbs, then each herb's dosage should be reduced by half or a third.

Ready References

www.ars-grin.gov/duke

Chapter 9: Antiviral Culinary Herbs & Recipes

Many culinary herbs have wide-ranging therapeutic benefits, and my research enables me to recommend them with confidence. There are actually so many healing (as well as tasty) culinary herbs that you have a wide selection from which to choose. You should know, however, that using a small amount of a single herb in your food will do very little to protect you from the flu or strengthen your immune system. You need to use a number of different culinary herbs each day for them to be an effective part of your bird flu survival plan.

In this chapter, I will discuss different ways of getting what I call a "medicinal daily dose" of these special herbs. For the maximum benefit, they need to be as fresh as possible. Dried herbs, especially if they have little smell or taste, may be old and exhausted and therefore they have little therapeutic value. Many of the culinary herbs you'll read about are listed as having antiviral activity in a major scientific textbook. Ref (1). Others are listed in a U.S. government database. Ref (2).

The number of antiviral compounds in some common culinary herbs are

- Common oregano — 22
- Thyme — 19
- Rosemary — 18
- Fennel seeds — 16
- Coriander — 15
- Marjoram — 14

These particular herbs, as powerful as they may be in fighting the flu, might not even be the best antivirals in the herb family, as many herbs have not been extensively tested. What this does show, however, is that ordinary kitchen herbs contain many known therapeutic compounds, including some with antiviral activity, and they are worthwhile flu preventives if you use them as recommended in this chapter.

For all culinary herbs I suggest you start with low quantities, as tastebuds need to adjust. At the same time, I am suggesting larger doses than recommended in most cookery books because for flu prevention you need more than a pinch of herbs — just don't use so much that your whole meal tastes bitter or unpleasant. Some herbs in this chapter may cause side effects (i.e. garlic may upset the digestive tract), in which case you might want to try tiny quantities occasionally or avoid it completely. If anything irritates your body it is not good for *you*.

NOTE: For pregnant women I suggest using only tiny quantities of herbs, rather than trying for therapeutic doses. As a general guideline, this means a pinch of mixed herbs per meal or a few fresh leaves finely chopped into a salad. If you're using herbal powders to make teas, I suggest that you mix them to a paste in water first because dry powders can irritate the throat. When you add powdered herbs to food, make sure they are thoroughly mixed through the food.

Three really important culinary herbs to strengthen the immune system are ginger, garlic and turmeric.

Ginger

For colds and flu it is best to use fresh ginger root because it is the essential (aromatic) oil in ginger that contains the antiviral actions. The easiest way to get an anti-flu effect is to grate fresh, uncooked root into your food or make a tea. Laboratory studies have confirmed the antiviral activity of ginger oil. Ref (1) & Ref (2).

Recipe for ginger tea

1-2 teaspoons grated fresh ginger root
1½ cups water

Bring to boil in a small saucepan; then simmer for about five minutes with the lid on. Turn off the heat and leave stand for a few minutes. Strain and drink — you can add stevia or honey to sweeten but do not add sugar or milk. It is better tolerated after food and I suggest 1-2 cups daily. You can change the quantity of ginger according to your taste. If you have leftover ginger tea, use the water when cooking rice, vegetables, soups or casseroles.

Ginger in cooking

Add raw grated ginger root into foods such as stir-fries and casseroles and remember to do this *near the end of the cooking time*, otherwise the aromatic compounds will be lost. I suggest starting with about ½ teaspoon per meal per person and then up to 2 teaspoons daily about three times weekly.

Other ways of using ginger

Powder, tablets and liquid extracts are available and a therapeutic intake of dried ginger is 2-4 grams daily.

NOTE: People taking anti-coagulant drugs or suffering from bleeding disorders should check with their doctor before taking ginger. Ginger liquid extract may cause upper digestive upsets, such as belching.

Garlic

Laboratory and animal studies confirm garlic's antiviral effects. Ref (1). There are 39 sulphur compounds in garlic and these are primarily responsible for the antiviral activity, which means that if garlic is completely deodorised it will ***not*** help to prevent or treat the flu. It is known that garlic can increase natural killer cell activity and enhance some specific immune cells. Researchers say that garlic may be a promising candidate as an immune modifier. Ref (2).

Odour-reduced garlic with caraway and vinegar

500 grams (17.5 ounces) garlic cloves

1-2 tablespoons crushed caraway seeds (antiviral and helps reduce garlic odour)

500 ml (16.6 ounces) apple cider vinegar.

Peel garlic cloves. Pack the garlic loosely into two 500 ml glass jars, sprinkling over the caraway seeds. Fill the jar with apple cider vinegar so that the garlic and caraway are completely covered. Seal with a firm lid, label and date. This is my version of aged garlic and it will last for more than two years. I find that it is less reactive for those with sensitive digestive systems and less odorous. Use in cooking on top of grills or in casseroles and roasts. It may also be used as a marinade or in salads. I suggest about ½ teaspoon per person to begin with, perhaps increasing to 1-2 teaspoons — which is the dose I have about 2-3 times each week.

Other ways of using garlic

Garlic is available as pastes and powders for use in cooking, and generally I suggest about ¼ teaspoon per serving, per person, initially. You can use a garlic crusher and squeeze a small segment (clove) of garlic over a salad or add up to a clove to your juicer if you are making a vegetable juice.

You can also buy garlic tablets, capsules and liquid extracts. I recommend enteric-coated tablets for most purposes. (Enteric-coated means that the tablet passes through the stomach intact and does not get broken down until it reaches the intestines, where it gets absorbed and consequently causes little breath odour.)

NOTE: Do not use garlic if you are taking blood-thinning medication. If you routinely use large quantities of garlic, stop 10 days before surgery. Do not use if it upsets your digestive system. If breath odour is a problem - try sucking a spirulina tablet after the meal or chewing some caraway seeds.

Turmeric

Turmeric is a spice derived from the rhizomes of curcuma longa, a member of the ginger family. Turmeric is one of the spices in curry powder. Turmeric is listed in a number of authoritative texts as having antiviral activity. Ref (1).

Curry powder recipe

2 tablespoons each of powdered turmeric and ginger

2 teaspoons powdered chilli

1 tablespoon each of cumin, cardamom and coriander (these herbs may be varied according to your taste and their availability).

The curry is much tastier if you buy seeds and chunks of dried herbs and grind them into a powder as required. I have a small electric coffee grinder that I use solely for herbs. After grinding put all the ingredients in a dark glass jar, seal and shake thoroughly to combine. Use a dark jar (or a light-proof container) because turmeric in particular degrades in the light. Label and date — remember the fresher the better.

An easier option is to buy a curry powder or curry paste. Read the labels. Use curry powder in mixed cooked vegetables or meat and chicken dishes. With cooked dishes, add the curry in towards the end of the cooking time. First, mix the powder to a paste in cold water and then add more water, so that it is easier to mix through the food. I like my food hot and spicy, so I add about ½ teaspoon per cup of food, but I suggest that you start with ¼ teaspoon per cup if you're not used to curries.

Other herbs, including garlic, may be added according to your family's tastes, but if you add too many herbs this will reduce the curry effect. I often add in some thyme, fennel and mustard powder. If you want a curry flavour but less heat, reduce the ginger and chilli and add one or more tablespoons of fenugreek powder.

NOTE: Some people are sensitive to hot spices. If anything irritates your mouth, throat or digestive tract it is not good for ***you*** and should be avoided. There are plenty of other herbs and foods that provide antiviral activity.

Easy lentil and barley curry

2 cups brown/green lentils
2 cups whole barley
2 onions
2 vegetable stock cubes
Curry paste or powder (quantities depend on your taste and the hotness of the curry — start with about ½ teaspoon per cup of dry ingredients)

Soak overnight 2 cups of lentils in 4 cups of water. Next day, put the soaked lentils in a pressure cooker. Add the whole barley and finely chopped onions, plus 4 more cups of water. Add the vegetable stock cubes and stir. Bring to pressure and cook at a moderate heat for 30 minutes. Stir in the curry and leave stand for five minutes before serving. If you don't have a pressure cooker or microwave, cook until the lentils are very soft — about 1 hour. If you use whole barley it will stay very chewy. If you use pearl barley it requires only about 10 minutes cooking in a pressure cooker. I don't add the curry at the beginning because it tends to stick to the bottom of the cooker and lengthy cooking reduces the herb's therapeutic effects. This is a very basic recipe — you could substitute the barley for whole rice and the lentils for chickpeas or other beans, although these need soaking and take longer to cook than lentils. Optional extras include tomatoes and fresh or dried herbs. Serve with a topping of plain acidophilus yoghurt and chives, together with separately cooked vegetables or salad. Serves 6-8 people.

Other ways of using turmeric

Good-quality turmeric gives a wonderful yellow colour to cooked dishes, but a disadvantage is that it has a bitter taste by itself. Use it sparingly. For instance, about a teaspoon is sufficient for two cups of cooked rice (or a stir-fry) for four people. Turmeric and its isolated compound, curcumin, are available in tablet form and liquid extract. Medicinal doses are high, up to four teaspoons of powder daily, but in the context of flu I recommend it as a preventive, using it as a culinary herb at about one teaspoon three or four times weekly.

NOTE: Aside from the rare possibility of an allergic reaction, there are no cautions relating to a dosage of up to one teaspoon in food per person four times weekly.

Other infection fighting culinary herbs

- Coriander
- Rosemary
- Thyme
- Cinnamon
- Mint
- Horseradish
- Cardamom
- Marjoram
- Oregano
- Cloves
- Sage
- Fennel & aniseed
- Hot chilli
- Basil
- Tarragon
- Nutmeg

Infection Fighting Herbal Combinations

To get an infection fighting effect from culinary herbs on a long-term basis you need to find a simple way of using at least some of these herbs every day. One way to do this is to:

- Select about six common culinary herbs that you have not included in your curry powder (see my recipe under turmeric). For example: dried thyme, sage, oregano, fennel, basil and tarragon.
- Put about two tablespoons of each of these into a dark-coloured, airtight jar and shake the jar so that the herbs are mixed together.
- Put a label on the container in case you forget the contents, and leave the container on the kitchen bench. If it's in a cupboard you won't use it when you are busy!
- When you are cooking vegetables, rice, casseroles or any savoury meal, simply add ¼ to 1 teaspoon (per person) of the mixed herbs towards the end of the cooking time.

If you don't want the actual herbs in the meal, you can buy a tea infuser — a small stainless steel container with holes — and fill it with dried herbs and leave it in the bottom of the saucepan while the food is cooking. This will only work if you have a reasonable amount of fluid in the saucepan. You will then get the flavour and some of the "goodness" of the herbs without the bits and pieces. (Strain and keep this water in the fridge to add to something that you cook within the next day or so, then you'll get extra nutrients and compounds from the food and herbs.)

This system of combining herbs saves you from handling many containers of herbs. And even if you grow fresh herbs, there are going to be times when you can't be bothered collecting them. Many of my meals are very "herby" because I may use dried herbs when cooking, plus a handful of freshly picked herbs to cut finely over the food when it is served. I do this frequently with parsley, basil, oregano and chives because they're easy to grow.

An even easier system is to buy a container of mixed herbs from your supermarket. You will find a list of contents on the label. Remember to keep it handy and use it regularly. I don't have rules about which herbs go with particular foods, although I tend to use a little cinnamon or clove with apples, and hot chilli and tarragon with dried beans.

Good herbal combinations for adding to Asian meals include coriander, ginger, cardamom, aniseed, cumin and mustard. Again — and I can't stress this enough — I add these toward the end of the cooking time because if you cook the herbs for too long, you lose much of the essential (aromatic) oil content into the air. It is these aromatic oils that contain much of the antiviral activity.

Information on Different Culinary Herbs

Coriander

Coriander is surprisingly powerful as an infection fighter. When you first use it, you may find the taste peculiar, so use very small quantities and gradually increase to about ½ teaspoon per person, per serving. I buy the seeds to grind and mix into curries, or to add to rice and Asian meals in particular. Some recipes tell you to fry the seeds in oil at the beginning of the recipe. I disagree, as this damages the therapeutic effect of the seeds. Coriander can be tricky to grow as it goes to seed readily, but seeds and powder are widely available. Try to use some at least twice a week.

Oregano

This herb is also surprisingly potent as an antimicrobial to fight infection. It is often used in Italian meals, but I use it freely in many types of cooking. Oregano is easy to grow and is a vigorous ground cover. I harvest some leaves at least two to three times a week and chop them finely into salads or use them over any cooked foods.

Rosemary

Rosemary has very good antiviral activity. Ref (1). It is very easy to grow, but the leaves are quite leathery and not convenient to use. If you don't have it growing you can buy it fresh or you can buy it in powered form. When I prune the plant I strip the leaves, put them in bottles and cover the rosemary with vinegar. This preserves the rosemary and draws out the active compounds from the plant. Then I use the vinegar in salad dressings. (You can use any of your garden herbs in this way and if you have the time, you can strain the fluid and then steep more herbs in it so that the herbal vinegar becomes more potent.)

Most people think of rosemary as the herb that goes with lamb. But you can also put the fresh leaves into a tea infuser so you get the flavour into soups or other cooked dishes. Another way to use this herb is to simply tie a small bouquet of rosemary and place this into the saucepan. This way, you get the aroma while the food is cooking, but when the food is done the leaves can be easily removed.

Baked fish with herbs

Lay fish fillets on a bed of fresh rosemary leaves in an ovenproof dish. Cover the fish with slices of tomato, then more rosemary. Over the top add a little soy sauce plus a sprinkle of vinegar or lemon juice. Then cover the dish and bake in the oven for about 30 minutes at 180 degrees Celsius (356 degrees Fahrenheit). The rosemary camouflages the fishy smell, provides flavour and adds immune-boosting benefits. Remove the rosemary before serving, but use all of the juice. You can use any combination and amount of fresh herbs in this way, but if you have dried herbs only, limit yourself to a total of four to five teaspoons.

Another way of using fresh rosemary leaves is to stuff them inside a roast chicken or place the leaves in the baking dish during cooking. Again, discard the leaves. Other fresh herbs, such as oregano, can be used in this way, as can combinations of any herbs that you have growing.

Thyme

Thyme has antiviral effects (see page 91) and is easy to grow but somewhat fiddly to use in cooking because you have to strip the tiny leaves from the woody stems. You may find it easier to buy powdered thyme and use it in the combination recipes I have already discussed. **NOTE:** If you eat woody pieces of plants or leathery leaves (such as rosemary and bay), these can get stuck in the throat or even the intestines!

Sage

Common sage is traditionally used for sore throats and fever. Sage can prevent the harmful oxidation of fats — so it is useful to add to meat dishes. Laboratory studies confirm that sage has antibacterial and antiviral activity. Ref (1). Sage is easy to grow and the leaves can be finely chopped and added to salads and cooked meals, including baked goods.

Sage tea

This tea is good for fevers and excess perspiration. Place 5-10 grams (10 grams equals one-third of an ounce) of the dried cut herb in a large glass jar (or twice the quantity of fresh leaves). Add 1 teaspoon crushed fennel or aniseeds (optional). Add the juice of one lemon. Pour over about 450 ml (15 ounces) tepid water. Cover and leave stand in the fridge overnight. Strain, and drink cold in 3-4 divided doses, flavoured with fruit juice. This is a high daily dose and would be taken for about a week.

NOTE: Do not use sage oil internally. Aside from small quantities occasionally in food, do not use sage as an oral remedy during pregnancy or if there is a history of epilepsy or seizures.

Cinnamon

Cinnamon has antiviral activity and it is a useful addition to formulas for respiratory infections because it improves the taste of the remedy. You can mix cinnamon powder into cooked apple, using about ½ teaspoon of cinnamon per serving for therapeutic purposes. As a general culinary herb, if you add too much the food tastes bitter. I use cinnamon in baked rice pudding, homemade bread and biscuits.

Antiviral cinnamon muffin recipe

1 cup buckwheat flour (or substitute)
½ cup self-raising wholemeal wheat flour (or substitute)
½ cup blackcurrants
½ cup sultanas
½ cup small walnut pieces
1 cup soy milk (or substitute such as coconut)
1 green apple, peeled and grated
3 teaspoons cinnamon or clove powder (or 50/50)
1 tablespoon olive or Niulife coconut oil (for greasing the muffin tray)

Combine all the dry ingredients. Add the soy milk and mix thoroughly. Spoon the mixture into the well-greased tray. Sprinkle the apple and cinnamon evenly over the tops of the muffins. Bake for 30 minutes at 180 degrees Celsius (356 degrees Fahrenheit). Makes 12 "mini" muffins.

Fennel and Aniseed

These two herbs have a long history of use as medicinal respiratory remedies, as well as being popular culinary herbs and teas because of their lovely flavour. I usually buy the seeds and grind them as needed to add to one or more of the combination formulas given at the beginning of this chapter — which means that I am having them two to three times a week. All plants in this family, including angelica, chervil, cumin, dill, lovage and parsley, have some antiviral activity. Dill is often suggested in fish recipes and parsley grows very easily, even in containers. Italian parsley may be used as a vegetable and both forms of parsley may be added liberally to salads and cooked meals rather than simply putting a few sprigs on the side of the plate for decoration.

Mint

Most edible and herbal mint plants have some antiviral action. If you are not fond of hot mint tea, use the leaves liberally for decoration and aroma in iced herbal teas, together with crushed ice, fruit juice or slices of fruit. The smell of fresh mint leaves in drinks is quite pleasant even if you don't like mint teas. I like to use finely chopped fresh mint leaves in salads, but you can buy it dried and add to any dried herb combination for general use in cooking. Peppermint and spearmint often grow rampant in the garden, so it's best planted in its own position.

Chilli

Chilli is one of my favourite herbs and is directly useful for the flu because it has antiviral activity. It clears the nasal passages and sinuses and it induces sweating, which is nature's way of cooling you down. Chilli is commonly added to foods that are hard to digest, such as beans. I recommend about one teaspoon per meal for six people to begin with, but remember that nature does not make plants uniform — some batches of chilli will be stronger than others. If you use fresh chilli, make sure that it is very finely chopped. If you use chilli powder, make sure it is mixed thoroughly with moist food — otherwise the powder can irritate the throat. Herbalists use liquid extracts and chilli capsules. (See the curry recipe under turmeric at the beginning of this chapter.)

NOTE: Hot chilli should be considered a herb and not a food. Enormous quantities of chilli (10 percent of the dietary intake) are harmful and some people cannot tolerate even tiny quantities, so use all hot spices wisely.

Horseradish

Horseradish is one of nature's best decongestants and has some antiviral and antibiotic effects. As a culinary herb, it is commonly used as a paste and served with cold meat. Mustard is similar to horseradish and is useful with meat because it aids digestion.

Basil

Holy basil is a traditional Ayurvedic herb that has been used for colds, flu and reducing fevers. This herb has been tested and found to have antiviral and antibacterial effects. The plant is sold in many nurseries, but some Indian people tell me it is not the same as "tulsi," the sacred basil plant grown in India.

In any event, it grows well all year round and I have used both the flowers and leaves extensively for many years in cooking and in salads. Common sweet basil is a seasonal plant that grows readily in warm seasons and is best used as finely cut fresh leaves with tomatoes or mixed into salads.

Also, cardamom, tarragon, marjoram and nutmeg are all good culinary herbs that are not generally used medicinally, although there is some evidence that they have mild antiviral actions. Cardamom has a wonderful flavour and smell, and I think it improves any herbal combination that you make up. Tarragon is somewhat bitter tasting, while marjoram tastes similar to oregano but not as powerful. Nutmeg causes nausea at high doses, but I find that a little freshly grated nutmeg goes really well added to spinach, together with some goats' cheese.

Most people's immune systems, and most meals, will be helped by a more liberal and regular use of culinary herbs. There is plenty of evidence to support their anti-flu and immune-strengthening benefits — and what better way to protect your health than enhancing the taste of your favourite foods.

Ready References: www.ars-grin.gov/cgi-bin/duke/activity.pl

Chapter 10: Aromatherapy with Antiviral Effects

Aromatherapy is basically the art of using essential oils for therapy. In this case, we will be looking at oils with antiviral actions. Essential oils are distilled out of plants and are very highly concentrated, so you should never use them as oral remedies or around the eyes. Essential oils are also known as aromatic or volatile oils, because they have distinctive and powerful aromas and they evaporate in heat.

Most oils derived from culinary herbs will have antiviral activity because it is the essential oil that provides most of the antimicrobial effects.

The herbs covered in this chapter have been laboratory tested specifically for antiviral activity — they show activity against flu viruses or other viruses in the same broad category as influenza.

NOTE: Some people are sensitive to aromas and to anything concentrated applied to their skin. If you are a first-time user of any essential oil, always test it first before breathing it in or using it as a remedy. Essential oils penetrate the skin and enter the bloodstream and it takes somewhere between 30 and 90 minutes for this to happen. I suggest that you put one drop of an oil on the inside of your elbow and then wait about two hours to see if you get any adverse reactions before using it therapeutically.

Lemon Oil

The essential oil of lemon is derived from the leaves of the lemon tree; the aroma is pleasant and relatively mild. The aroma is usually well tolerated even if you are feeling sick, making it useful as part of flu treatment. From the scientific evidence, lemon leaf essential oil has the highest concentration of antiviral activity. Ref (1).

Using lemon oil

- **Inhalation:** Put three drops of essential oil into a cup. Pour over (add) hot water but be careful not to burn children and do not use in children under the age of eight. Place a towel around the cup and over your nose while you breathe in the fumes. (You could also put a paper bag over the cup and cut a hole in one corner.) This inhalation is surprisingly powerful. A simpler variation is to use a few drops of oil on a handkerchief (placed under your pillow at night), in a vaporiser or in an aromatherapy oil burner.
- **Chest rub:** Add six to 10 drops of lemon essential oil to 50 grams of vitamin E cream (or any ointment base — coconut oil is lovely to use). Gently massage about a teaspoon of the cream into the chest — this is best done at bedtime.

Other citrus oils, such as lime and orange, contain antiviral compounds. I like to use lime oil in my car, either adding it to a damp cloth when cleaning the interior or simply sprinkling a few drops on the floor. It's refreshing and helps clear the respiratory system.

Tea Tree Oil

The essential oil of this Australian plant has a long history of use as an antiseptic and is classed as a broad-spectrum antimicrobial. Ref (1). Tea tree oil affects viruses before they penetrate cells, which means that it may be a useful flu preventive.

Using tea tree oil

If you put one drop of oil on your toothpaste you will amazed at the antiseptic strength. Put one drop of oil under your nose to clear nasal passages. As a mouthwash and gargle, add one to two drops of oil to ½ cup tepid water. Stir the oil into the water before using. Tea tree oil can also be inhaled like lemon oil (see above).

Eucalyptus Oil

Eucalyptus is a well-known antiseptic and has very similar antiviral effects to tea tree oil. Ref (1).

Using eucalyptus oil

Put one drop of eucalyptus oil under your nose to help with breathing and to relieve sinus congestion. An option is to buy an inhaler from a pharmacy or health food store, as these often contain eucalyptus and other oils and are convenient to use. Steam inhalations of these oils are good for reducing nasal and sinus blockage/congestion. Remember that your respiratory system is your first line of immune defence and when you get congestion this allows for a build up of viruses and bacteria.

Using eucalyptus oil or tea tree oil as a household antiseptic

Add six to 10 drops to your washing machine, or onto a damp cloth for household cleaning. Pour about ½ a capful down the kitchen sink and in the toilet bowl — your family will also be breathing in the antiseptic vapour.

Chapter 11: Antiviral Drugs and Vaccines

You will have noticed that up until now, my focus for surviving a flu pandemic has been on (a) building a strong immune system, (b) the steps you can take to avoid a bout with bird flu, and (c) the antiviral foods and herbs that will help increase your body's resistance to this potential killer. I've virtually ignored vaccines and the antiviral drugs mentioned so frequently in the mainstream press — and there is a good reason for that.

There is not a vaccine available today that will prevent you from being infected with H5N1 bird flu.

It's possible that the leading antiviral drugs now on the market — specifically, Tamiflu and Relenza — will not be as effective in treating bird flu, at least in all cases, as a lot of people are claiming or hoping.

To really control a bird flu pandemic, vaccines and antiviral drugs will be needed in much larger quantities than current planning will cater for.

According to the U.S. National Institute of Allergy and Infectious Diseases, each person needs to be given 90 micrograms of killed bird flu vaccine virus, in two doses four weeks apart, for adequate immunity. This is around 12 times the amount of virus normally needed for an effective flu vaccine. The world's existing vaccine-manufacturing technology and infrastructure would not be able to meet the demand for bird flu vaccine — the output would be way below what is needed for a global pandemic.

NOTE: Antibiotics will not help you if you have the flu. Antibiotics do not kill viruses, including viruses that cause the flu. Antibiotics kill bacteria, and their only effective use as regards the flu — and that is any type of flu — is for fighting the secondary, bacterial infections you may come down with as a result of having the flu. Using antibiotics when not required can make them less effective when they are really needed.

Vaccines

Vaccines, and not antiviral drugs, are the key to stopping a bird flu pandemic, but as I just noted there is currently no vaccine to protect humans against the bird flu virus that keeps showing up in poultry and to date has killed about 50 percent of the relatively small number of people who've been infected. On top of that, it's unlikely that an effective vaccine will be available in adequate quantities until after a bird flu pandemic is well under way.

To back up for a second, at present there are two types of flu vaccines: the flu shot, which uses a dead virus and is given with a needle, and a nasal spray that uses a live, weakened virus. With either method, antibodies will develop about two weeks after the vaccination, and it is antibodies that will protect you against the flu should you be exposed. For a vaccine to work, it must trick the body into creating those antibodies — your own natural defence against the flu. For a vaccine to be effective, the virus used to make it must match the strain that is actually infecting people.

When you have a strain of the flu like H5N1 that is still changing and has not yet mutated to a point where it can easily infect humans … well, what this means is that any sample of the current H5N1 virus that's used in a vaccine today will not be an exact match for the virus that may cause a future bird flu pandemic. And if it is not an exact match, the flu-fighting antibodies it will prompt your immune system to create won't be nearly as effective as they could be.

One option is to just wait until a pandemic begins before making a vaccine. The problem with this approach, though, is that it would likely be a minimum of three months, and perhaps as long as nine months or even a year, until sufficient amounts of an effective vaccine was available. At that point, given the speed at which an easily transmitted form of bird flu would spread, having a bird flu vaccine — no matter how well it worked — could be largely irrelevant.

Realising that this wait-and-see attitude toward developing an H5N1 vaccine would likely result in tens of thousands — or more — deaths should a pandemic occur, governments and researchers are working together to come up with a vaccine solution. For instance:

- The United States government has teamed up with a private pharmaceutical company to develop nasal sprays that might not only be effective against the H5N1 bird flu strain, but a number of other genetically unique flu strains as well. In all, researchers hope to develop at least 16 different vaccines, with the idea that one might be an exact or very close match to any pandemic flu virus that arises. Human testing on the first of these vaccines is already under way.
- The La Jolla Institute for Allergy and Immunology is conducting three major research initiatives to attack the influenza virus — and says all three may be applicable to the H5N1 virus. The research, which is fairly complex, involves taking a protein common to all influenza A viruses — including bird flu strains — and using that protein to immunise mice that are genetically engineered to produce human antibodies. In laboratory testing, the antibodies created in the mice bound to several different flu strains, including H5N1 bird flu. This means infected cells would be recognised by the antibody and destroyed by the immune system. Clinical testing in humans is the next step.
- An Australian company has begun human testing with a vaccine that it says would be effective against H5N1 bird flu virus in humans — unless the virus undergoes major genetic changes. "The mutation that would make it spread from human to human … is probably not enough to render the vaccine ineffective," said a spokesman for CSL Ltd.
- Several biotechnology companies are at work on a new and quicker way of making flu vaccine, one that involves injecting people with just a few DNA genes extracted from a flu virus, rather than the traditional process of using chicken eggs to manufacture vaccines. Human trials may begin in 2006, though any mass-produced DNA-based product is still probably several years away.

Yet, even if an effective vaccine for bird flu was already available, current global production capacity falls far short of the demand expected during a pandemic. What many people fail to realise is that flu vaccines are a biological product and not something that can be created with chemicals — vaccines cannot be cranked out overnight or made by just mixing together a bunch of ingredients in a large vat. For the traditional flu vaccine, viruses are grown in hens' eggs, then killed and purified before being made into the vaccine. This takes months.

It's the time involved in making flu vaccines that has prompted some scientists to suggest doses be divided during a future pandemic so that more people can be vaccinated with a weaker vaccine, one that will minimise, but probably not prevent, the flu. Unlike ordinary flu, where a lot of people choose not to be vaccinated, I suspect that in the event of a bird flu pandemic, almost everyone would want protection. Who knows, maybe divided doses would be the best or the most practical solution if/when a pandemic occurs...which is just another good reason for making sure your immune system is as strong as possible.

Antiviral Drugs

Antiviral drugs are a key component of most government and public health plans to combat bird flu. But at present, there are only two drugs — Tamiflu and Relenza — that health officials think might be effective against whatever mutated form the H5N1 bird flu virus might eventually take.

Both drugs are designed to fight the flu in the same way: by interrupting the ability of the flu virus to replicate in the body.

The flu virus invades your cells and turns each cell into a virus factory to make more viruses inside the cell. Once made, these new viruses need to escape from the cell so that they can go out and invade more of your cells. The new viruses use a protein enzyme called neuraminidase to cut themselves free from the cell in which they were made. Relenza and Tamiflu are "neuraminidase inhibitors," because they inhibit the enzyme needed for a virus to cut itself free from the cell.

Bird flu is a particularly nasty virus, killing its victims indirectly by unleashing an extremely severe inflammatory response that causes massive tissue damage and blood vessel leakage in the lungs. It's not uncommon — as previously mentioned — for a bird flu patient to literally drown in his or her own lung fluids. Scientists are also investigating drugs that target the lungs to reduce tissue damage, inflammation and respiratory distress. But for now, the standard recommendation is that Tamiflu and Relenza be used as the first line of bird flu defence.

In particular these antiviral drugs are recommended for:

- All high-risk patients with influenza. This would include the very young, the very old and those with co-existing diseases such as asthma or other lung diseases, cardiovascular diseases and immuno-compromised individuals.
- All persons with severe influenza.
- If there were adequate supplies the antiviral drugs could be used to protect people with known exposure to someone infected with the bird flu virus in a pandemic.

Tamiflu (Oseltamivir)

Tamiflu has been widely publicised for some time now as mankind's best hope for surviving bird flu and many of my patients have told me they think it can cure bird flu. In reality Tamiflu can only make the illness less severe.

There is some credible evidence, however, that the H5N1 bird flu virus may be resistant to Tamiflu — at least in the dosage that up until now was considered adequate.

A December 2005 report in the prestigious *New England Journal of Medicine* reported that Tamiflu-resistant forms of the H5N1 bird flu virus were found in two Vietnamese girls who died despite taking the drug. The report focused on eight patients who were treated for proven infections with the H5N1 bird flu virus at the Hospital for Infectious Diseases in Ho Chi Minh City between February 2004 and January 2005. All of these patients were given Tamiflu when they were admitted to the hospital, which varied from two days to eight days after onset of their symptoms. They were prescribed the usual dose of Tamiflu tablets, which is 75 mg twice daily for five days. Unfortunately, four out of the eight patients died.

It's important to note here that Tamiflu, like many antiviral drugs, is most effective if administered within 48 hours after symptoms are first noticed. Not all eight patients met this deadline. Yet even so, two of the girls who died developed a Tamiflu-resistant form of the H5N1 virus, which has prompted some doctors to suggest that the recommended dose may be too low. Doses of medicine that aren't strong enough to kill viruses or bacteria can instead allow them to mutate and re-emerge in a slightly different and more aggressive form.

Health officials are still recommending that Tamiflu be used to treat bird flu patients, although some are saying we need to use higher doses for longer periods of time. Further studies will determine the safety of a higher dosage, and hopefully the effectiveness as well.

Relenza (Zanamivir)

Relenza was developed years before Tamiflu; however both drugs were released on the American market in 1999.

In August 2005, the *Lancet Journal* published an article showing that:

- Relenza was just as effective as Tamiflu, but had fewer side effects
- The flu virus was less likely to become resistant to the antiviral effects of Relenza, as compared to Tamiflu

Relenza has not demonstrated the resistance that Tamiflu has, and may be effective in conditions where Tamiflu is not. The *Lancet Journal* recommended that governments stockpile both Relenza and Tamiflu. The company that developed Relenza is now developing a new long-acting neuraminidase inhibitor which is currently in clinical trials. At present Relenza is only available in an inhaled form, although an intravenous version of the drug is being developed.

How effective is Relenza?

Relenza reduces the duration and severity of the flu, but like Tamiflu it is most effective if taken within 48 hours of the onset of symptoms. It has been shown with the regular flu virus that if you take Relenza as a preventative (before you catch the flu infection), you may not get any flu symptoms at all.

NOTE: In the event of a pandemic, do not take any antiviral drugs or antibiotics without your doctor's advice. This is most important, as premature use of any antiviral drugs or antibiotics could (1) make the virus more resistant to drugs or (2) make the drugs less effective, if and when you really need to take them.

A point of reassurance as regards both Tamiflu and Relenza is that there is no sign that the H5N1 virus that's now circulating among wild birds and poultry has become resistant to either of these drugs — despite the Tamiflu resistance that occurred in the two Vietnamese girls. Both antivirals may well play a very valuable role should a pandemic occur.

Antiviral Drugs and the Future

The Australian government is stockpiling supplies of Relenza. They placed their order in December 2005 and it will take until April 2007 to fill. Australia is one of the best prepared countries and has Relenza coverage for 40% of its citizens.

The World Health Organization recommends that countries stockpile at least one course of either Relenza or Tamiflu for 25% of their population. The rationale here is based on the **hope** that both drugs would be effective for **prevention** and **treatment** during the first stage of a pandemic, whilst waiting until an effective vaccine was developed.

Warnings for Drugs and "Miracle Cures"

Before we leave the subject of drugs and the flu, there are a couple of things you need to be aware of:

- First, know that dishonest people out for a quick dollar are making unproven and fraudulent claims that certain products and therapies will provide 100 percent protection against bird flu. To date, warnings have been issued to at least nine different companies for trying to sell bogus flu products. In the words of one public health official, "The use of unproven flu cures and treatments increases the risk of catching and spreading the flu, rather than lessening it, because people assume they are protected and they aren't. I consider it a public health hazard when people are lured into using bogus treatments based on deceptive or fraudulent medical claims." The message here is two-fold: "Buyer beware" and "If it sounds too good to be true, it probably is."
- With all of the recent publicity about bird flu, and with it being common knowledge that antiviral drugs are in short supply, many people have been talking to their doctors and shopping around trying to stockpile antiviral drugs. If you buy Tamiflu or Relenza outside of normal channels, there's a chance they may be counterfeit. Fake shipments have already been intercepted.
- Finally, even if you have one of these antiviral drugs on hand, you may take it at the wrong time or in the wrong dose. That will offer you little protection and increase the likelihood that the virus will become resistant to the drug. If you get symptoms of a respiratory infection, without a flu test and doctor's examination, it's very hard to know if you have influenza; thus if you used up your supply of drugs you would not have them when you really need them. For these reasons experts do not recommend that individuals stockpile personal supplies of antiviral drugs.

Flu viruses are great survivors. To be a survivor yourself, begin strengthening your immune system now, use common sense precautions to avoid the flu, and only take drugs and medications when absolutely necessary and when prescribed by a doctor.

Survival Plan Summary

"An influenza pandemic of even moderate impact will result in the biggest single human disaster ever — far greater than AIDS, 9/11, all wars in the 20th century and the recent tsunami combined. It has the potential to redirect world history, as the Black Death redirected European history in the 14th century." — Michael Osterholm, Director, Center for Infectious Disease Research and Policy

I'd say that the above statement not only sums up the potential for worldwide death and destruction that a bird flu pandemic presents — but should also put you in the frame of mind to begin your own survival preparations now.

In summary the four key components of a well-thought-out survival plan are:

1. Keep your immune system strong
2. Stockpile things you need to survive
3. Use basic infection control procedures
4. Stay aware of the current situation

1. Keep Your Immune System Strong

Your immune system is your best weapon against a fatal infection from the H5N1 bird flu virus or, indeed, any severe infection. At the very minimum, I suggest the following to keep your immune system strong and healthy:

- Take regular supplements of vitamin C, selenium and zinc – see chapter 6
- Consume a raw juice at least three times a week – see page 76
- Include the Super-immune foods in your regular diet to strengthen your immune system – see table page 58
- Use culinary herbs with antiviral properties regularly in your food – see chapter 9
- Take flu-preventive herbs — the best ones are olive leaf extract, ginseng, echinacea and thyme. Olive leaf elixirs can be used for children and there are some that contain added thyme & vitamin C.
- Don't smoke cigarettes.

2. Stockpile Items You Need to Survive

In the event of a pandemic, supply lines will be disrupted, stores and supermarkets may close and there may be shortages of many necessities and fresh produce.

Here is your survival checklist:

- A juice-extracting machine and a manual citrus juice squeezer (that does not need electricity) in good working order.
- A supply of fresh raw vegetables and fruits to eat and juice; better still, start your own organic vegetable garden. You can grow herbs in pots on the veranda, balcony and windowsill as well as in the garden. Make up several large bottles of our antiviral raw juice recipe (see page 77) to store in the freezer. Frozen, it will last for years!
- A supply of extra vitamin C tablets, capsules or powder (kept in a cool place in airtight containers).
- A supply of zinc lozenges – see page 54
- Bottles of tea tree oil and lemon oil and an aromatherapy oil burner.
- A supply of food (food supplies are likely to become limited during

a pandemic) – choose canned food high in protein, such as fish (salmon, sardines, tuna, etc.), canned or dried beans, whey protein powder, rice, sea salt and honey. This will make it easy to keep up your protein and energy intake without the effort of much cooking.

- A supply of fresh citrus fruit (lemons, oranges and limes). Make up several litres of freshly made citrus juice to store. It will last for years in the freezer!
- An extra refrigerator with a large freezer to store and keep the virus-fighting foods and juices fresh and active.
- A supply of antiviral foods such as canned coconut cream, cold pressed virgin coconut oil, canned tomato paste (goes well with beans), dried medicinal mushrooms, walnuts, etc. – see chapter 7
- Bottled water or a water filter; better still, get a rain water tank.
- Povidine iodine liquid to sterilise objects and drinking water plus a supply of antiseptic soap.
- A supply of face masks.
- A supply of disposable thin plastic gloves.
- A supply of goggles for you and your family.
- A supply of tissues and paper towels.
- A supply of antiviral herbs — the best ones are thyme, olive leaf and elder.
- A bottle of antiviral vinegar to strengthen the immune system; this is suitable to freeze (for the recipe see page 80).
- A supply of onion antiviral cough remedy; this is suitable to freeze (for recipe see page 66).
- A good first aid kit with two accurate thermometers, analgesics (such as paracetamol and ibuprofen) and a good supply of any prescription medications you and your family require, etc.
- Torches and plenty of batteries
- A radio that can be battery operated or a crank radio
- Candles and matches
- Extra cash in case banks shut down
- Disposable knives, forks, spoons and plates
- A manual can opener
- Extra canned or dried food for any pets you might have
- An "I can survive anything" attitude.

3. Use Basic Infection Control Procedures

In a pandemic, use the strict procedures I discussed earlier to control infection in your own home and to protect yourself when venturing outside. – see pages 49-50. At the very least, these measures will reduce the amount of virus that gets into your body, so that the initial assault of bird flu will be lessened. The greater the number of flu viruses in your body, the greater the inflammatory response will probably be, with more risk of complications.

4. Stay Aware of the Current Situation

Watch and read the news and, if possible keep a broadband connection to the Internet so you can be the first to know when bird flu strikes your area. This will enable you to learn of any new breakthroughs in vaccines or antiviral drugs that may help you survive a pandemic. Also:

- Register for the Google link on bird flu updates www.google.com/alerts?hl=en

- Know the website address of your government health department – you can check out their preparedness plan and become aware of new breakthroughs. Useful Australian website addresses are -
  www.health.gov.au/internet/wcms/publishing.nsf/Content/phd-pandemic-plan.htm
  www.health.nsw.gov.au/infect/pandemic flu.html

- Make a list of the symptoms of bird flu so you can recognise the first signs of infection in you or your family members (see page 37)

- Have a good relationship with your local doctor or medical centre so that your medical history is known — check to see if your doctor does intravenous vitamin C for severe flu infections

- Keep lines of communication open with your doctor

- Know the address and contact details for the best hospital near you that has good facilities and an intensive care unit

You do not need to panic or live in a heightened state of fear and anxiety – but you need to remain aware of the events happening around you. If a pandemic arrives in your area, panic will only make things worse and hard to control. Lack of knowledge and lack of preparedness lead to panic. If you already have a survival plan and have stockpiled the things you will need, the risk of panic is greatly lessened.

Most health experts on the front lines of the pending war against bird flu do not have an optimistic outlook. The risk that the H5N1 bird flu virus, or some other form of bird flu, will become efficient at sustained human-to-human transmission will remain with us for as long as flu viruses continue to circulate in birds. This will likely be for years and years to come.

We all hope that the worst never happens, but the wise among us will be prepared in case it does.

FINAL NOTE: This book is NOT intended to replace or be a substitute for the care and supervision provided by your own medical doctor. At all times you should remain under the care of your doctor. The suggestions and advice in this book are to be followed only in conjunction with your regular medical care. I am not saying that I have the cure for bird flu — this book is designed to be used as a survival guide and is not a substitute for medical treatment for any flu infection.

Pandemic Awareness for Businesses and Corporations

Businesses will play an important role if an influenza pandemic occurs and they need to be informed if they wish to protect the health and safety of their employees and reduce the adverse impact upon the economy and the community. They should use all the information and resources available to them to form a plan to cope with an influenza pandemic

Important things to consider in such a plan are -

- Identify a pandemic coordinator or a team within the company structure with specific roles for preparedness
- Prepare a plan to enable employees to work and communicate with each other from home
- Assess logistics for staggered shifts, job sharing and training for overlapping roles and multi-skilling of employees
- Assess possible impact of a pandemic on company financial status, product lines and production sites
- Educate workers on how to find reliable and up to date pandemic information and help from the government health department, community public health and local hospital.
- Educate workers with information in written form about influenza – cover the signs and symptoms of influenza, how it is transmitted, how to protect oneself and family and how to avoid panic and incorrect information (such as myths, rumours and unproven or dangerous treatments)
- Assess employee access to and availability of health care services during a pandemic
- Plan for employee absences during a pandemic and establish policies on non-punitive sick leave and when an infected person who has recovered can return to the workplace
- Encourage and document annual influenza vaccination for employees
- Educate employees on good hygiene, infection control procedures, and personal protection kits for use in the workplace and for travel to potentially affected areas

- Provide the equipment and supplies to reduce the risk and spread of infection – such as paper towels, tissues, masks, antiseptics, alcohol wipes, gloves, goggles, plastic lined rubbish bins
- Assess local community resources for obtaining vaccines and antiviral drugs
- Educate staff that there must be immediate exclusion of co-workers with symptoms of respiratory infections or exposure to others with proven infections – they must be given immediate mandatory sick leave.
- Develop policies to restrict work necessitated travel of employees to affected areas or countries and to evacuate employees working in affected areas when an outbreak begins
- Collaborate and communicate with other businesses, chambers of commerce and pharmacies in your local community – you may learn from each other and improve the response effectiveness of your local community.

Planning needs to take into consideration that in any given community an influenza outbreak is expected to last six to eight weeks. This would be followed by at least two new pandemic waves.

For more information visit -

http://pandemicflu.gov/plan/tab4.html
http://pandemicflu.gov/plan/businesschecklist.html
http://www.webmd.com/content/article/113/110741.htm

Glossary

Acute: In medicine, this relates to an illness or a reaction that is sudden, severe and of short duration, such as the flu.

Antibodies: Proteins that are produced by immune cells to neutralise and destroy viruses

Antigenic drift: Antigenic drift refers to small, gradual changes that happen continually over time, to produce new virus strains that may not be recognised by antibodies to earlier flu strains.

Antigenic shift: Antigenic shift is an abrupt, major change that produces a new virus not seen in humans in many years, if ever. This new virus can spread easily and cause serious disease since there is no natural immunity.

Antioxidant: Substances that help protect human cells from the damaging effects of oxygen free radicals.

Antiviral: Any substance, natural or manmade, that is capable of reducing the ability of a virus to survive, infect and multiply.

Aromatherapy: The use of fragrant essential oils extracted from herbs, flowers and fruits for medicinal and health promoting effects.

Avian: relating to birds – see bird flu

Bacteria: Any of a group of single-celled microorganisms that live in soil, water, organic matter or the bodies of plants and animals. Many types of bacteria are essentially harmless, while other types of bacteria cause illness that range from pneumonia to meningitis.

Bird flu (avian): Bird flu, or avian influenza, is a group of different flu viruses that mostly infect birds, but will occasionally infect other species — most notably, humans.

Carotenoids: A group of pigments ranging in colour from light yellow to red that are widely distributed in plants and animals. The best known is beta carotene, which is found in carrots. Cartenoids are antioxidants.

CDC: The Centers for Disease Control and Prevention (CDC) is one of the 13 agencies of the U.S. Department of Health and Human Services. Since it was founded in 1946 to help control malaria, the CDC has been at the forefront of public health efforts to prevent and control infectious and chronic diseases.

Cytokine storm: This is an extremely aggressive inflammatory reaction of the immune system to an infection. If it occurs in the lungs, they may fill up with fluid to the point you can't get oxygen into your lungs and thus into your blood. Even artificial ventilation in an intensive care unit may be useless against such severe lung inflammation and mortality rates are very high.

Decoction: The result of boiling a herb or plant into a concentrated form to extract its flavour and essential ingredients.

Extract: Extracts are made according to specific pharmacopoeial directions, and come in concentrated form. Alcohol is often used in herbal extracts to draw out the therapeutic components and act as a preservative.

Flavonoid: Flavonoids are a class of water-soluble pigments found in many plants. While not labelled as essential nutrients, many of these compounds serve as antioxidants and are anti-inflammatory and immune balancing.

Free radicals: These are highly reactive molecules that are produced within the body and can destroy cells and cellular compounds. Free radicals are produced by pollution, stress, trauma and infections amongst other things.

H5N1: H5N1 is the scientific name of a strain of avian influenza. At present, it is primarily caught from direct contact with infected live poultry and from touching surfaces or objects that are contaminated with infected raw poultry meat, poultry faeces or saliva.

High pathogenic: At very high risk of causing or being capable of causing a severe disease.

Immunity: The quality or state of being able to resist and overcome disease, particularly infectious diseases such as the flu.

Inflammation: A physical response that can cause bodily tissue to redden, grow hot, swell and be painful as a result of illness, infection or injury.

Influenza: By definition, influenza — or "the flu" — is an "acute and highly contagious respiratory illness caused by viruses and characterised by mild to severe illness and, at times, death."

Influenza A viruses: Influenza type A viruses can infect people, birds, pigs, horses, seals, whales and other types of animals, though wild birds are the natural hosts for these viruses.

Interferon: A type of protein produced by immune cells to help the body overcome infections by blocking viruses.

Lactoferrin: Lactoferrin is a whey compound (whey is a by-product of cheese making) that seems to enhance the body's ability to fight viral infections.

Legumes: Legumes are beans, peas and lentils; they have some benefit to the immune system because they contain lignans and isoflavones that are known to have antiviral properties.

Lignans: Lignans are basically fibre-rich foods — the highest sources are whole ground linseeds (flaxseed), pumpkin seeds and berries. All whole grains contain lignans, but refined grains do not. Studies indicate that lignans can exert some worthwhile antiviral effects.

Low pathogenic: At relatively low risk of causing or being capable of causing a disease.

Lymphocytes: Lymphocytes constitute 20 to 44 percent of the body's white blood cells and are the main means of providing the body with immune capability.

Macrophages: These special immune cells ingest and destroy the body's foreign invaders; for example, viruses and bacteria.

Microorganisms: Tiny "bugs" or germs; these are visible only under a microscope. They can cause minor to major infections. Bacteria and viruses are two examples.

Natural killer cells: White blood cells that do battle with viruses and tumour cells. They also produce components that stimulate immune function, but are less active when you are severely stressed.

Naturopath: A healthcare provider who avoids drugs and surgery and emphasises the use of natural agents such as air, sunshine, water, fruits, vegetables, herbs and massage.

Nitric oxide: A gas that is normally produced in the human body and is thought to play a role in strengthening immunity.

Oxidation: A process that occurs when a substance combines with oxygen.

Pandemic: An influenza pandemic, which is simply a worldwide epidemic, occurs when a new flu virus to which no one has any natural immunity (antibodies) appears in humans, causes serious illness, and is able to spread easily from person to person and from country to country.

Phagocytosis: The ingestion and destruction of microorganisms by white blood cells and macrophages.

Probiotics: These are friendly bacteria (mostly found in yoghurt) that keep unhealthy germs in your intestines at a low level.

Relenza: Relenza (Zanamivir) is an inhaled antiviral drug that has been approved to treat people for uncomplicated influenza virus infection. Clinical studies showed that for the drug to be effective, patients needed to start treatment within two days of the onset of symptoms.
RNA: RNA or ribonucleic acid is part of the genetic makeup of a virus.
SARS: Though similar to the flu — including its early symptoms — SARS, or Severe Acute Respiratory Syndrome, is a severe form of pneumonia that originated in China in 2002. It was caused by a coronavirus, one of a group of viruses responsible for respiratory illness in humans and diseases in animals.
Sodium ascorbate: The sodium salt of vitamin C that's used in a sterile solution when vitamin C is given in liquid form through a vein.
Stevia: Stevia is a South American herb and natural sweetener that is calorie-free and to which many health benefits have been attributed. Stevia is 150 to 400 times sweeter than sugar.
Tamiflu: Tamiflu is an antiviral drug in tablet form. Like Relenza it works by attacking the influenza virus and stopping it from spreading inside the body.
T cells: A specialised immune cell, which is a major component of the immune system; T cells are very helpful in combating viruses, fungi and bacteria.
Tofu: Tofu, also known as soybean curd, is a soft, cheese-like food made by curdling fresh hot soymilk with a coagulant.
Vaccine: A solution containing infectious agents that is either injected or inhaled to artifically build up your immunity (antibodies) to a particular infection or disease.
Viruses: Viruses are very small particles — approximately one-millionth of a centimetre (2.54 cm equals 1 inch) in size — that are responsible for a wide range of illnesses, from AIDS, glandular fever, warts, cold sores and colds to hepatitis and the flu.
WHO: The World Health Organization is the United Nations' specialised agency for health. It was established in 1948 to help all of the world's people to attain the highest possible level of health. Health as defined by WHO is a state of complete physical, mental and social well being.

Bibliography – Scientific References & Evidence

Spanish Flu

Ref. 1. http://Itc.smm.org/buzz/blog/1918_flu_virus_recreated

Ref. 2. Robert B. Belshe, The Origins of Pandemic Influenza – lessons from the 1918 Virus, The New England Journal of Medicine, 353; 21 Nov 24, 2005, www.NEJM.ORG

Ref. 3. Kobasa D, et al, Enhanced virulence of influenza A viruses with the haemagglutinin of the 1918 pandemic virus. Nature 2004; 431:703-707

Echinacea

Ref. 1. http://sunsite.sut.ac.jp/pub/academic/medicine /alternative-healthcare/herbal-references/Herb-Research-Foundation.

Ref. 2. Forum Immunologie, 8: 1-8: 1992.

Eight out of nine 'medical trials' treating upper respiratory infections demonstrated that echinacea decreases the severity and duration of the infections. Journal of Family Practice, 48: 628-35: 1999.

Archives of Pediatric and Adolescent Medicine, 158; 217-221: 2004.

American Journal of Clinical Nutrition, 72; 339-47: 2000 (page 12).

New England Journal of Medicine, 353; 341-8: 2005.

Ref. 3.

- A university laboratory made the test echinacea product but the laboratory processes were not be in accordance with specified manufacturing procedures set out in herbal pharmacopoeia - and the American Botanical Council report that it does not equate with commercial echinacea products.
- The dose used in the trial was unclear and presumed by the American Botanical Council to be the equivalent of 900 mg per day of the dried root, which is somewhat less than the amount I would use for prevention and about a third of the dose I prescribe for treatment. The WHO lists a daily dosage of 3 gram (3,000 mg) daily of echinacea root.
- The trial used US college students; they had a particular type of cold virus inserted into their nostrils and they were confined to a hotel room for a week. Apart from the reality that a week is not enough time to build up the immune system, this procedure does not mimic what happens in the real world. And, would you be stressed if confined to a room for a week? Or, were the students 'living it up' or overusing room

service - and unwittingly causing physical stress? All types of stress weaken the immune system. *International Reviews of Neurobiology*, 52; 93-131: 2003.

Ginseng - Known immune effects

Ref. 1.

- A scientific trial of 175 people tested ginseng at a dose of 100 mg twice daily for four months. After one month, an influenza vaccination was given. Blood tests showed that the ginseng group developed higher levels of antibodies after vaccination – which means enhanced protection against the flu. *Alternative Therapies*, 7; 104: 2001.
- Any major physical or mental stress is likely to depress the immune system. Over 20 studies (mostly animal) show that ginseng permits better toleration of various physical, biological, chemical or psychological stresses. This includes viral infections and exposure to radiation and poisons. *Bulletin of Experimental Biology and Medicine*, 101; 627-9: 1986.
- Laboratory studies showed that ginseng significantly increased two important immune functions - natural killer cell activity and antibody-dependent cell cytotoxicity (the ability of antibodies to kill infected cells). *Immunopharmacology*, 35; 229-35: 1997.
- In patients with chronic bronchitis, a standardised ginseng product activated alveolar (lung) macrophages indicating a specific potential for preventing infections in the respiratory system. *International Journal of Immunotherapy*, X, 21-4: 1994
- Animal studies show that ginseng enhances immune cells (B and T-lymphocyte activities) and increases production of the immune chemical interferon. *Planta Medica*, 50; 462-5: 1984.
- Dr DVC Awang reviewed the immune effects of ginseng and found that the herb increased and activated spleen cells, activated immune cells and increased IgG (an antibody that fights infections) In: Janick J, ed, *Perspectives on new crops and new uses*, ASHS Press, Alexandria, VA, 1999. *British Journal of Pharmacology*, 134; 1663-1670: 2001.

The above is a selection from the many published scientific papers available in English; there is much more information available throughout Asia – and the research is ongoing.

Ref. 2. Journal of the American Geriatric Society, 52; 13-19: 2004.
Ref. 3. Canadian Medical Association Journal, 173, 1043-8: 2005.
Ref. 4. Antiviral Research, 50; 223-8; 2001.
Ref. 5. British Journal of Phytotherapy, 2; 61-71: 1991.

Hypericum (St John's Wort)

Ref. 1. Antiviral Research, 13, 313: 1990.
Ref. 2. Medicinal Research Reviews, 15; 111-19: 1995.

Astragalus

Ref. 1. 'Boosting Immunity with herbs', http://sunsite.sut.ac.jp/pub/academic/medicine/alternative-healthcare/herbal-references/Herb-Research-Foundation.

Elder

Clinical trials have confirmed the benefit of elder:

- A standardised elder syrup at a dose of 2-4 tablespoons daily gave a complete cure from influenza B within two to three days in nearly 90 per cent of cases compared to six days in the placebo group. Blood tests also confirmed a much better outcome in the elder treated group. *Journal of Alternative & Complimentary Medicine*, 1; 361-9: 1995. It was also reported that elder was active against seven human influenza viruses and three animal viruses.
- Elderberry syrup at a dose of 15 ml four times daily allowed influenza A symptoms to disappear four days earlier than placebo. *Proceedings of the 15th International Conference on Antiviral Research*, Prague, March 2002.
- Several strains of influenza virus were inhibited in laboratory studies and researchers subsequently reported that an elder extract trial on humans seemed to offer an efficient, safe and cost-effective treatment for influenza. *Journal of International Medical Research*, 32; 132-40: 2004.
- Based on human blood tests, elder was shown to activate aspects of a healthy immune system. *Israeli Medical Association Journal*, 4; 919-22: 2002. It may be useful not only against influenza but also for immunodepressed cancer or AIDS patients.
- A combination of elder, St. John's wort and soapwort was active against influenza A and B. *Phytotherapy Research*, 4; 97: 1990. A number of other laboratory studies confirm the effectiveness of this combination, including a study combining it with a pharmaceutical (an amantadine derivative) on the reproduction of influenza virus strains A/H1N1 and A/H3N2. *Acta Virologica*, 37; 258-64: 1993

Olive leaf

Ref. 1. *Life Science*, 62; 541-6: 1998.
Ref. 2. http://www.phytotherapies.org/monograph_detail.cfm?id=153
Ref. 3. http://users.ren.com/wussery/olivel.html
Ref. 4. http://www.bastyr.edu/academic/botmed/herbs.asp?HerbId=148869264
Ref. 5. Posit Health News, 17; 12-4: 1998
Ref. 6. Biochemical and Biophysical Research Communications, 307; 1029-37: 2003
Ref. 7. Antiviral Research, 66; 129-36: 2005.
Ref. 8. http://scholar.google.com/scholar?hl=en&lr=&q=%22olive+leaf%22+antiviral

Licorice

Ref. 1. Microbiology and Immunology, 26: 535-9: 1982.
Ref. 2. Licorice Monograph, *The Review of Natural Products*, February 1998.

Thuja

Ref. 1. *British Journal of Phytotherapy*, 2; 182: 1992.

Pau d'Arco

Ref. 1. Jones K, *Pau d'Arco*, Healing Arts Press, Rochester, USA, 1995. (857 references).

Ginger

Ref. 1. *Journal of Natural Products*, 57; 658-62: 1994.
Ref. 2. Bradley PR, ed., *British Herbal Compendium*, Vol. 1, British Herbal Medicine Association, Bournemouth, UK, 1992.
Recommended reading: Paul Schulick, *Ginger: Common Spice & Wonder Drug*, Herbal Free Press Ltd, Brattleboro, VT, 1996. (This reference lists 477 compounds in ginger, and gives 356 references)

Garlic

Ref. 1. Phytomedicine, 2; 73-91: 1995
Ref. 2. Journal of Nutrition, 131; 1075S-79S: 2001.
Ref. 3. Advances in Therapy, 18; 189-93: 2001.
Ref. 4. Phytomedicine, 6; 325-330: 1999.

Turmeric

Ref. 1. *American Surgery*, 64; 47-51: 1998.

Rosemary

Ref. 1. *Food Chemical Toxicology*, 34; 449-56: 1996.

Sage

Ref. 1. ESCOP *Monographs on the Medicinal Use of Plant Drugs*, 1997.

Culinary herbs

Ref. 1. Charalambous G, ed., *Spices, Herbs and Edible Fungi*, Elsevier, Amsterdam, 1994.

Ref. 2. Dr Duke's Phyto-chemical and Ethno-botanical Databases, http://ars.grin.gov/cgi-bin/duke.

Lemon Oil

Ref. 1. Dr Duke's Phytochemical and Ethnobotanical Databases, http://www.ars-grin.gov/cgi-bin/duke/activity.pl.

Tea Tree Oil

Ref. 1. *Journal of Applied Microbiology*, 99; 170-5: 2000.

Eucalyptus oil

Ref. 1. *Pharmazie*, 56; 343-7: 2001.

Mushrooms

Ref. 1. International Journal of Immunopharmacology, 14; 971-7: 1992.

Ref. 2. Review of Natural Products, Monograph, May 1997 (44 references)

Ref. 3. *British Journal of Pharmacology*, 139; 289-98: 2003. (48 references)

Nutrients to strengthen the immune system

J. W. Lampe 'Health effects of vegetables and fruit,' American Journal of Clinical Nutrition, 70 (suppl): 475S-90S, 1999; summary p. 484-5

Whey

Ref. 1. http://www.msstate.edu/org/fsfa/Vol1/2-Pihlanto.htm.

Ref. 2. http://www.cals.wisc.edu/media/news10_99/whey_Etzel.html.

Ref. 3. *American Journal of Clinical Nutrition*, 82; 69-75: 2005.

Yoghurt

Ref. 1. Meydani et al, Immunologic effects of yoghurt. American Journal Clinical Nutrition 2000, 71:861-72

Ref. 2. American Journal of Clinical Nutrition, 74: 833-9: 2001.

Medicinal herbs

Ref. 1. http://www.ars-grin.gov/duke

Jassim SAA, Naji MA, 'Plant products as antimicrobial agents', *Clinical Microbiology Reviews*, 12; 564-82: 1999. (148 references)

Cowan MM, 'Novel antiviral agents: medicinal plant perspective.' This researcher concludes "The traditional use of some of the medicinal plants for the treatment of infectious diseases of viral origin, therefore, is justified." (253 references), *Journal of Applied Microbiology*, 95; 412-27: 2003.

http://scholar.google.com

Selenium

Dr Margaret Rayman, Dietary selenium; time to act, British Medical Journal, Vol. 314, 387, Feb 1997

Nelson HK, et al. Host nutritional selenium status as a driving force for influenza virus mutations. FASEB J 2001;15:1846-1848

http://www.surrey.ac.uk/SBMS/ACADEMICS_homepage/rayman_margaret/

http://scholar.google.com/scholar?hl=en&lr=&q=selenium+antiviral

www.laucke.com.au/health/SeAVEffects.htm

Zinc

www.coldcure.com/html/hand_2.html

http://scholar.google.com/scholar?hl=en&lr=&q=zinc+antiviral

Antiviral drugs

Hayden F, et al. Neuraminidase Inhibitor Susceptibility Network position statement: Antiviral resistance in influenza A/H5N1 viruses. Antiviral Therapy 2005; 10 (8):873-7

De Jong MD, et al. Oseltamivir resistance during treatment of influenza A (H5N1) infection. New England Journal Medicine, 2005 Dec 22; 353 (25):2667-72

Index

emergency diseases watch hot line

If you notice sick birds or other sick animals who are possibly infected with the bird flu virus, it is important to contact the relevant authority

The Australian government has established a hotline for reporting exotic diseases in animals; this includes avian influenza

The phone number to call is

1800 675 888